The Nutrition Nanny

Maria Burns

Pinocular Press
Copyright © Maria L Burns, 2012
All rights reserved

To every child of God: may you play more and eat less sugar!

*While every effort has been made to ensure its accuracy, this book's contents should not be construed as medical advice. Everyone's health needs are unique to the individual and the author shall have neither liability or responsibility can any injury caused or alleged to be caused directly or indirectly by the information contained in this book. The concepts, ideas, and suggestions in this book are not intended as a substitute for consulting with your physician.

Table of Contents

Acknowledgements

Thank you to my Creator. It is in You that I find myself and to You whom I belong. Dad, thanks for being my rock, sounding board, and the amazing person you are. I am so grateful to my mom for making sure I played outside everyday and teaching me to love broccoli. Thanks to all my brothers for adding so much fun and laughter to my life and to my friends for their support and encouragement. A very special thank you to my two beautiful and amazing grandmas for your endless love and feedback. You are the most amazing role models a gal could ask for. Lastly, thanks to all the people who have let me experiment with their diets and all the awesome nutritionists and doctors who wrote the books that led to those experiments.

Chapter 1
Peek Through My Pinoculars

"Health is not everything, but without it, everything else is nothing." Doctor Bernard Jensen

Have you ever stared deeply into the core of your.... favorite fruit? If you look closely enough, you might just find that the answers to all of life's problems are right there, encased in the apple of your eye. It holds seeds of new beginnings, the promise of life, and nourishment for the body, mind, and spirit. Close your eyes for a moment and imagine the stress in your life being peeled away.... health concerns, family issues, and life's disappointments all becoming additions to the compost pile.

One of the many times that I was staring deeply into the (pine)apple of my eye, I was lost in wonder by all the amazing food that God put on the earth. Seriously, how did He dream that flavor up AND make it good for me? I suddenly wished I could see nutrition from His perspective. What would He have to say about food today and all the health problems that are results of poor diets?

It was that moment I suddenly understood nutrition's connection to God. He was the very first nutritionist. He created the nutrients and the unique packages that contain them, designed to give life and health to the creations He loves.   Wanting to understand nutrition from His perspective, I decided to fashion a pair of pinoculars (pineapple binoculars) and peek at nutrition from the perspective that God is the ultimate nutritionist.

The Path to the Pinoculars

I wandered into the world of nutrition when I noticed its powerful impact on everyday life, and therefore on my job as a nanny. Growing up as the only girl of my parents' eight children, I was quite familiar with childcare and the kitchen by the time I was eight. I used to be miffed when I was stuck inside on kitchen patrol while my brothers worked outside with my dad on Saturdays.   As I grew up, though, I came to love cooking and taking care of kids. I discovered that the kitchen was a rather magical place; people, particularly men, could mope in crabby with a chip on their shoulder and saunter out with a smile and murmurs of satisfaction.   Kids could collapse into chairs, all played out, and within a half hour, feel ready for round two. I realized that the kitchen was all about life support.

When I wasn't in the kitchen, I spent most of my free time playing outside with brothers and friends, whether it was in the summer sunshine or the winter snow. My childhood is the reason that I nannied for two years in college, and after graduating, I opted to au pair in Germany and then become a professional nanny out in California instead of applying for a job in the area of my degree-finance. I loved being a kid and have loved being around kids all my life.   It is the freedom of children from inhibitions, cynicism, and worry that makes them special and their energy, curiosity, and laughter that make them so enjoyable to be around.   Throughout my years of nannying, I began to notice a trend that disturbed and saddened me. I saw kids that lacked those freedoms, energy, and lightheartedness. I saw kids whose childhoods were tainted with all sorts of worries that should not be on the radars of children.

There are moments in life that can be pinpointed as the start of something, be it a journey, a change of heart, or a pursuit of a dream. The moment that ultimately set this book in motion happened long ago. I was helping Kylie; a cute five year old, awesome big sister, and spectacular conversationalist, get ready for a birthday party. As she tried on outfit after outfit, her frustration increased. Finally, on the verge of tears, she threw the eighth outfit on the floor, exclaiming, "Nothing looks good on me because I am so fat!" I almost burst into tears. That a child her age should have to deal with self-consciousness and worry because of her appearance is heartbreaking.

That moment would revisit me often throughout the years, until it sparked a desire in me to rid those experiences and issues from as many children's lives as possible.

It was in Germany while I was an au pair that I became extremely interested in nutrition. It was impossible not to notice the differences between the health and happiness of families and children there compared to the US. Families spent a lot more time together. They ate more meals together and spent time engaging in activities that did not include the television. Children were happier, more active and better behaved, and I was surprised to see respectful teenagers that enjoyed and chose to spend time with their parents on weekend nights. It was also impossible not to notice the differences when it came to food. Smaller grocery stores, simpler meals, and less of an overlap of popular culture and food were all characteristics that contributed to less of a focus on eating than is present in the US. After moving out to California, I studied nutrition at the Natural Healing Institute while nannying professionally, which stoked my interest and led to an interesting hobby.

Dissatisfied with the proposed solutions to obesity that came from current clinical trials and research, namely the "eat a Balanced diet" and "enjoy all foods in Moderation" approach, I began to backtrack in time. I ordered all kinds of nutritional books from the 1950's, 60's, 70's, and 80's. What I found absolutely fascinated me. The changes to the food and culture back then were the beginning of the obesity crisis that is present today. Reading about the changes in people that doctors and nutritionists were seeing and their opinions on the causes of those changes, was eye-opening, explanative, and intriguing. I learned an incredible amount from the documentation of these doctors' hands on experience with individual patients. They did not rely solely on laboratory research or scientific studies to prove their points: their proof was in their patients' results. These old school nutrition books laid out case after case of people that were struggling with all the problems that are now at the core of the health crisis: depression, excess weight, lack of energy, and dissatisfaction with life. Case after case, these doctors were restoring their patients' health using nutrition.

Reading about the changes that these doctors made to their clients diets supported my hunch that balance and moderation are not the proper solutions to help people overcome diet related disease. Not once, in about twenty books, did I hear the suggestion to use the sickening substances (sugar, refined flours, etc) in moderation. The word I heard over and over was eliminate. These doctors were telling their patients to eliminate the substances that were causing the problems. Complete elimination led to restored health and renewed interest in life.

Over the course of five years, nannying for five different families, I saw more and more instances of children dealing with problems that stemmed from their diets. Sneaking food, refusing healthy food, obsession with food, and low self-esteem because of weight were traits that I saw often and were clearly linked to diet. Issues that I began to notice were connected to diet were school performance, overall attitude and energy levels, the ability to manage emotions, interactions with siblings, and obedience to superiors. The more I learned about nutrition as I nannied, the more I saw the connection between children's diets and the the kind of children they were. Learning about food's physical and mental influence on people while seeing its practical application everyday at work was a powerful combination that confirmed and reinforced what I was learning day after day.

The more I learned though, the more frustrated I became. Witnessing malnutrition in families, and seeing both the problems and solutions in families related to food without the ability to help the situation began to really bother me. Never because the parents did not care about the health of their children, it was most often due to the misconceptions that abound when it comes to nutrition-a product of

4

advertising and media. Much of what I was learning is in contrast to broadly accepted standards of nutrition and I certainly didn't fault the parents for following the advice of those standards. Some families were open to change and wanted to become healthier, but it was often part of my job to feed children contrary to all that I had learned and believed. It was this frustration and my desire to help families who truly want to become healthier and happier that led to this book. It is my hope, that my journey and what I have learned along the way can help you to strengthen you and your family in body, mind, and spirit. I invite you to peek through my pinoculars and experience a perspective of nutrition that is the fruit of faith, observation in the lab of life, and the search for answers that have been lost in time.

Nutrition impacts your Mind just as much as it does your Waistline

The human body is a magnificent creation under brutal attack today. Its beauty, strength, and vigor are being slyly stolen away, and all the while we are told that the poisons responsible are not to blame. One in two Americans are expected to be obese by 2030. This impacts each and every one of us, but especially parents. With statistics like that, it is imperative to fight now for the health of your family, of your children, and of your future. No one is going to do it for you, and no one cares more about the health of your family than you. In order to avoid today's health epidemic from spreading into your home or to eradicate problems already in residence, a serious reevaluation of the status quo is in order.

Everything I have learned from my studies in nutrition, my experiences as a nanny, and my journey through life has brought me to a realization that I believe with every fiber of my being: the way you eat and the way you feed your family has a profound influence on all aspects of your life. It affects your thoughts, your sex life, how you spend your time, and your enjoyment of life. Chronic exhaustion, depression, anxiety, and lethargy are widespread today and are directly connected to the diet. Besides the impact that physical and mental diseases have on the individual, they also have a negative impact on family life. Malnutrition is so detrimental to the family that it is often a contributing cause to divorce and violence in our society. After all, how can a marriage be happy and healthy when the spouses are not happy and healthy? Because the extent to which malnutrition deteriorates both mental and physical health is massively underestimated, the possibility that it can damage a marriage is rarely considered.

In the 1960's, there was a psychologist named Cecelia Rosenfeld who saved many of her patients' crumbling marriages by correcting improper nutrition. While it might seem preposterous to think that food can be a factor when it comes to marital woes, the evidence is in reality. She documented case after case of marriages on the brink of divorce that were restored to health by nutrition.

The connection between mind, body, and soul is undeniable, and yet so much of today's health "knowledge" ignores that. A majority of experts today ignore the fact that what people eat affects their minds just as much as their bodies. Mental health issues are rampant and pills are given at the first sign of the blues, anxiety, or inability to concentrate. These pills simply treat symptoms, ignoring the cause, and often worsening the situation. Many mental health issues are simply manifestations of malnutrition. They occur because people are filling their bodies with toxins instead of food. Malnutrition hurts the brain as well as the body.

If a car that required 91 octane gasoline was filled with 87, it wouldn't be surprising if the car started having problems and stopped working efficiently. So it goes with the human vessel; when it is filled with the wrong kind of fuel, it is going to start having performance problems. The human body cannot be expected function as well on chemicals made in labs and processed junk as it does on real food. Just as muscles require protein, the brain requires nutrients to function properly.

Cutting through the "noise" of today's nutritional teachings

The plethora of theories, diets, and recommendations that exist when it comes food has made achieving good nutrition incredibly complicated and difficult. For every diet that tells you not to eat this, there are five more that say to eat that. For the normal person, this abundance of information and misinformation to sift through is overwhelming. Deciding what to put in your family's stomachs should not be so complex.

In the "War on Obesity" that is being raged, one of the most popular and most ineffective approaches is the "**BM**" approach that focuses on eating a **Balanced** diet with all foods in **Moderation**. The reasons for this are twofold. First, this idea has zero basis in reality. The "BM" theory has been around for more than a decade, with no visible results other than a 10% increase in obesity. If this approach actually worked, 36% of adults and 17% of children would not be obese, and an additional ⅓ of both adults and children would not be overweight. The second reason for the failure of this approach is the assumption that everything sold as food is actually food.

The "**BM**" theory claims that "all food types" can be part of a healthful diet. That claim is unsubstantiated though. Where is the evidence? Do the statistics for obesity, heart disease, cancer, and child diabetes in our country illustrate that junk can be part of a healthful diet?

What is a healthful diet? Is it one that simply keeps your BMI in an acceptable range? I think not. A healthful diet must go beyond that; a healthful diet supports life and keeps disease at bay. There is no way to include junk in the diet without an aftermath that reflects its addition. Laws of nature cannot be broken without repercussion. The question is not whether they will appear. It is when will they appear. Whether the consequences of malnutrition manifest in your 20's with depression, your 30's with diabetes or your 50's with cancer, they will appear.

The inability to translate the theory of "**BM**" to reality makes it useless. All the clinical trials and scientific studies that lead to the claims that junk can be part of a healthy diet lack practical application. Logically, it is peoples' overuse of, and therefore INABILITY to moderate junk that is responsible for the obesity epidemic today.

7

People do not decide that they want to eat more and gain weight. They don't open the box of cookies determined to eat every last morsel.

The **"BM"** approach claims that labeling food as good or bad, is simple minded and can cause people to reject nutritional guidance. Essentially, it says that the truth cannot be handled. It also endorses the use of "nutritive sweeteners" (the newest term for white sugar) as part of a "balanced" eating plan. Really? When along its demolition of Americans' health did sugar become worthy of being labeled as nutritive?

How is it that the battle cry for the "War on Obesity" is "balance and moderation?" Conquering the obesity epidemic is going to require something more extreme and simple than vague advice to "eat with awareness." Trying to achieve a diet of **"BM"** for yourself and your family is like a binge drinker trying to identify the perfect amount of drinks he can have before moderation is no longer possible.

Health professionals do not advise smokers who are at risk for lung cancer or already have it to smoke in moderation. They tell them to remove the substance responsible for lung cancer from their lives. People at risk for diabetes or obesity on the other hand are told to simply moderate their consumption of the problematic substances. Considering the fact that they would not have the problem to begin with if they were able to moderate their consumption, this advice seems to be the opposite of helpful.

So why is it that we are incapable of limiting what we put in our stomachs? Are two out of three Americans simply lacking the self-control to stop putting too much into their mouths? When someone tries to quit smoking and then caves in and lights a cigarette, what does that say about their self-control? Because we have been told how addictive cigarettes are, we understand the difficulty of breaking the habit. It is an unfortunate truth that there is an addiction of the same strength that is the culprit for people's inability to moderate how much they consume, which will be explored in chapter six.

Amidst all the vague dietary advice, busy parents are at an incredible disadvantage. Constructing a balanced diet that includes all "food types" includes addictive substances that are not really food. Many adults and most children do not understand the impact nutrition

8

plays in their lives, and considering everything that can be put into your mouth, it is easy to pick a diet based on taste.

The terms moderation and balance are extremely vague, which is a dangerous adjective in the realm of diets. I have seen intelligent, educated parents consider their children's diets balanced when they contain 200 grams of added sugar a day.

My years as a nanny showed me that all the mumbo jumbo presented as nutritional advice to parents is far too complicated. Eating in a healthy manner should not be rocket science; it should be simple.

Chapter 2
Foodtrition Fundamentals

" To be a true food, the substance eaten must not contain useless or harmful ingredients."- Dr. Herbert Shelton

Welcome to the concept of foodtrition. Simplicity is its backbone. Instead of focusing on making sure you get enough of the hundreds of nutrients while keeping other "items" in a vague "balanced" range, foodtrition takes an incredibly basic approach. It categorizes all the options that there are to eat into two categories: real food (food) and fraudulent food (fRood).

Food:
1. God's creations that consist of protein, carbohydrate, and fat used in the body to provide energy, and sustain growth, repair, and vital functions.
2. Does not contain elements that are harmful to your health or longevity.

fRood:
1. Fraudulent food
2. Contains ingredients that damage the body, prevent healing, or deplete energy.
3. Anything containing refined and/or processed sugars, flours, and grains.
4. Altered substances, that started out as food, but have been taken so far from their natural state that instead of contributing to health, they harm it.

Foodtrition:
1. Choosing only food, as close to its natural state as possible, to eat.
2. A diet devoid of fRood, chemicals and toxins.

Food versus fRood

Food	fRood
All vegetables	Anything containing refined sugars or corn syrup
All fruit	enriched/bleached/white flours
Nuts and seeds	soy products & anything containing soy (except for organic and fermented soy)

Food	fRood
Whole grains like oats, brown rice, quinoa, barley, millet, amaranth	Juice (except for fresh squeezed), soda, sports drinks,
poultry, meat, eggs, fish,	Anything containing hydrogenated oils
beans and legumes	processed snacks
cocoa	salad dressings, marinades,
whole grain flours	mayonnaise, sour cream, cream cheese
	pizza rolls, mozzarella sticks,
	Genetically Modified Organisms (GMOs)
	Anything containing MSG
	Items containing modified corn starch
	heavily processed dairy

fRood is tricky because it is such a poser. In the grocery store, clever packaging and marketing help disguise the fRood as food, even claiming that it is healthy. Ditching fRood is going to require that you ditch most things that come in packages from the grocery store. There are whole aisles that will no longer require your presence.

Foodtrition is so simple because everything you are eating supplies your body with nutrients and does not deplete them the way fRood does. It makes it simple because it is no longer necessary to stare at nutrition fact labels and try to make sure you aren't consuming too many trans fats or too much refined sugar or added sodium. This is because real food has none of those things. There are programs designed to teach children how to read food labels so that they can moderate how much junk they intake. I like the concept of teaching them the difference between food and fRood much more. It is easier to understand, keeps them healthier, and prevents them from developing fRood addictions. Teaching kids to count calories, sugar, fat, and sodium can also lead to eating disorders if the children become fixated on tracking their diet. When they eat real food, they don't need to count anything since their bodies will function properly. They will eat when they are hungry and only until they are full. Food does not cause overeating the way fRood does.

Whether your diet includes animal products is a matter of personal preference, lifestyle, and values. I believe that both vegan diets and paleo diets can be healthful if done correctly. If you do choose to include animal products in your diet, however, they should be as natural and free of hormones, processing, and additives as possible.

Slathered in sick syrup

The human body does not appreciate the tendency to cover food in sauces. Salad dressings, marinades, and gravies are usually loaded with two things: sugar and the bad-for-the-body types of fat. The sugar/bad fat combination is a killer combination. Literally, it will kill you. Timing is the only part of the equation that is not definite.

So(y) Evil

Often touted as an excellent source of protein, soy is overly processed, toxic, and filled with a type of estrogen that is not good for either sex. The high temperatures at which soy is processed denature it and make it indigestible. Over time, the type of estrogen that is present in soy builds up in the body and can lead to estrogen related diseases (like breast cancer, ovarian cancer, infertility, and painful periods). 90% of soy in the United States is also genetically modified.

Even if you don't drink soy milk or eat tofu, chances are that if you eat fRood, you consume quite a bit of soy. Processed foods are teeming with it in the form of soy oil, soy flour, soy lecithin, and soy protein. It is in baby formula, protein bars, granola bars, and cereal. Chips, crackers, salad dressings, marinades, and even whole wheat breads are loaded with it.

The only time that soy is okay is in small amounts when it is organic and fermented. Fermentation results in a product that the body is able to assimilate because it has been predigested.

Juice

Unless juice is fresh squeezed, there is no reason to include it in your diet. Juice has a high sugar content because all the fiber of the fruit has been taken out. Because juice has been pasteurized, all its enzymes and many of its nutrients have been killed. Many juices are not even 100% juice and are not much better than beverages like soda and sugary sports drinks. Whole fruit is the way to get your fruit fix and water is the way to hydrate.

fRood and your Family

The biggest hurdle to your family's health and happiness is overcoming the addiction that causes us to eat fRood instead of food. Health takes a back seat to taste in respect to what most people choose to eat. Eating primarily for enjoyment (based on taste preferences) radically disables wellness, happiness, and the ability to enjoy the rest of life (everything outside of eating). The biggest obstacle to your family's health and happiness is addiction to fRood.

Marketing and advertising are often people's source of information when it comes to their knowledge of nutrition. Just as a drug dealer is unlikely to tell you that the meth he is selling killed someone yesterday, companies selling fRood are unlikely to tell you that it is harmful to your health. They prefer to take the opposite approach and tell you that it is good for you. Cereal with soy protein, fruit snacks fortified with vitamin c, cookies loaded with nutrition, and breakfast shakes fortified with vitamins are all examples of fRood being passed off as healthy food choices.

The awesome news is that giving up fRood doesn't mean you have to starve your taste buds. In chapter fourteen, there are all kinds of recipes that will help you make the transition from fRood to food. From cookies to ice cream, muffins to pancakes, chocolate milk to hummingbird cake, you can still satisfy your sweet tooth, but instead of any guilt or fRood whatsoever, you will be filling yourself with nutrients that will make you vibrant, inside and out. And the more you eat wholesome foods, the more you will enjoy them, as your taste buds heal from the constant onslaught of poison they are so used to.

Although I am not an expert who has logged hundreds of hours in labs, studying various substances' effects on people, I have logged thousands and thousands of hours where the practical application of food lies. As a nanny who simultaneously studied nutrition, I got to see first hand, on a daily and extended basis, the role and effects that food and fRood have on children and families. I saw how their behavior changed according to what they were being fed, and I saw trends and patterns emerge throughout the long term care of 14 different children. As the woman of the house (kitchen) for my family, I have seen the awesome results that occur when a home transitions from fRood to food.

With all the health problems on the horizon that are facing your family, it is more important now than ever before to choose health for your family. If you don't decide that you want your children to have healthy, vibrant, and fulfilling lives and teach them how to achieve that life, they aren't going to learn. They don't learn at school; they are given fRood and sugary drinks there. In fact, the amount of sugar that children receive at school is staggering. In my years of nannying, I've seen kids receive soda as a reward for keeping their desk cleans, candy for snacks at after school programs as well as in their classrooms, and sugary junk at classroom parties. And then there is all the fRood that they are able to purchase in vending machines and in the lunch line. This occurs at public schools, private schools, schools on military bases, and even preschools.

The level of influence that nutrition and malnutrition have on lives is severely underestimated. Performance at work, quality of parenting, and achievement of goals are all impacted by what you choose to chew and swallow.

Everyone is born with inherent weaknesses and strengths courtesy of heredity. While these differ from person to person, fRood impacts everyone similarly in that it attacks weaknesses. Whether there is a history of acne, breast cancer, or depression in your family, fRood exacerbates the problems to which you are prone.

fRood is full of costs to our society. Besides the financial costs of diet related diseases, what about the opportunity costs of ideas, efficiency, and productivity at companies. fRood fueled employees are not going to perform as well as employees whose diets consist of real food. And the cost of that is immeasurable. The breakthrough ideas and creative solutions to problems that are nonexistent because employees don't have the proper fuel to produce them is definitely a cost to society.

As I share what I have learned about food, fRood, and family throughout the book, I hope that it resonates with you and that you find the inspiration, motivation, and faith, that it is possible to give your family the gifts of health and happiness.

Chapter 3
God's Garden

" More precious than gold is health and well being, contentment of spirit than coral." Sirach 30:15

The Chief of Nutrition (CON)

It is impossible to achieve an accurate understanding of nutrition while ignoring its genesis. Its very existence is based on the most important nutrient of all. Love is at the core of every apple and everything I learn about nutrition always brings me back to love. It was out of love that God not only created us, but also the food that nourishes us. Because He created us, He knows our bodies and what they need better than any scientist or nutritionist ever could. He is the Chief of Nutrition! That simple fact has many implications when it comes to eating. First, in looking at the foods that God created, it is a wonderful example of how awesome He is and how much love He has for us. He has wrapped every nutrient that our bodies need to thrive into beautiful and delicious packages in nature.

Viewing the culinary creations God has gifted us with makes one truth clear. God is almighty and no human mind can accomplish what He does, which is to create. That is why no man made fRood will ever be able to compare to what He has put in nature for us. No refined, processed, preserved, or copycat version will ever be able to nourish our bodies, minds, and spirits the way that God's fresh food does. The farther we take food away from its natural state, the more of God's wonderful gifts of love and life are lost.

Our bodies assimilate nutrients best when they are ingested in the original packaging of whole food. Because that packaging has been designed by the same Creator who designed us, it offers the highest quality nourishment available. The whole food package contains nutrients, enzymes, and fiber in ratios that work synergistically when eaten together. That synergy exists because of God's intimate knowledge and understanding of His creations. No amount of tweaking, combining, or modifying can result in more superior products than the food from God's Garden.

When whole foods are unwrapped and processed during their degradation to fRood, the synergy is destroyed and the end product holds significantly less nourishment and value than the original package. Then there is the matter of the destruction of nutrients throughout processing because of high temperatures and oxidation. Even when the fRood is "enriched", it cannot come close to equaling its former life, before its nutrients and synergy were pillaged in processing. The synergy of living, whole food is invaluable while "enriched" fRood contains nutrients (often of questionable quality) that are haphazardly added to a range of harmful ingredients to make a product appear healthy, although it is not.

Even if a piece of bread were to be baked with flour that had been "enriched" with every nutrient present in a red pepper, the red pepper would still be far superior to that piece of bread. The red pepper is a package straight out of nature that has not unwrapped, broken, put back together, and rewrapped into a different package.

Ninja Nutrients

Besides vitamins and minerals, food designed by God is brimming with hundreds of different phytochemicals that are flat out awesome. These super chemicals are responsible for the color of all

20

the food from the plant kingdom and have the most incredible and beneficial impact on our bodies. Antioxidants, catechins, proanthocyandins, terpenes, and xanophylls are just a few of the many classes of phytochemicals that detoxify the body, prevent cancer, and beautify the bod. Somewhat mysterious, there is much that remains unknown about these ninja nutrients. Everything that is known about them shows the extraordinary life support they offer. Even though no RDI exists for these them, they are essential if you want to enjoy health and happiness. My personal favorites are lycopene (I love the sun and this protects against skin cancer) and quercetin (improves stamina by increasing the blood flow).

Eating vibrant colored food from nature is one of the keys to thriving in life. Those vivid hues in fruits, vegetables, legumes, grains, and nuts signal the presence of the potent ninja nutrients that when ingested, immediately fight for your health. The expression, "add color to your life" is more than fitting when it comes to deciding what to eat. Eat a rainbow and discover the health and happiness at the end of it. The benefits they provide to the body number into the unknown, having an impact on everything from your toes to the crown of your head and from your skin to your internal organs.

Eating to Support your lifestyle

If an athlete was not eating adequate protein and his muscles started to deteriorate, the reason would be crystal clear. The solution would not be to label his active lifestyle as dangerous and unhealthy: it would be to support his lifestyle by eating an adequate amount of protein.

Nutrition in your life should be looked upon in the same way. A diet that supports the life you truly desire. Today it seems that our lifestyles conform to our diets. We resort to lethargic lifestyles because our diets do not support active ones. We shun the sun because of skin cancer, but ignore the influence that diet has on the situation. If you eat cookies and chips and sit in the sun, cancer is likely because your body is deficient in the nutrients it needs to allow you to spend time in the sun safely. Just like an athlete's consumption of protein allows him to safely exercise without damage to his body, eating the right kinds of food allows you to safely spend time outdoors in nature.

Instead of avoiding sunshine out of fear of wrinkles and skin cancer, perhaps the answer is to eat the food in God's garden loaded with the ninja nutrients that fight free radicals and ward off cancer. A diet rich in selections from that garden supports a lifestyle that can include sunshine and fresh air.

The sun is essential to life. Think of what would happen if you tried to grow plants without sunshine. They would not thrive. They would wither. It is the same for us. Sunshine delivers vitamin D, triggers the release of mood boosting endorphins, and can even speed up healing. We were not created to spend all our days cooped up in buildings. But we have to eat food that supports time in the sun.

It is ironic that despite the condemnation of the sun, billions of dollars are spent each year to mimic the effects that sunlight has on the body. Bronzers and blush for the face, highlights for hair, and sunless tanning lotions for the body are all products used to achieve the appearance of time spent in the sun. That is because the sun gives a beautiful and healthy glow to the body. It is interesting that it is the things in life that are healthy for the body that make it more attractive. Good nutrition, love, and exercise increase attractiveness. Perhaps the reason that the sun kissed glow is so beautiful is because sunlight lends elements to our bodies that we need.

Avoiding the sun because of skin cancer and aging concerns comes with an opportunity cost. What do you do inside instead of playing outside? Sitting on the couch in front of the tv or computer while munching on fRood is not going to save you from cancer or aging. fRood is full of toxic material that causes free radicals and cancer. A fRood based diet does not support life at all.

Garden of Love

When you eat a red pepper straight from a garden, you are receiving God's love, just as when you take in a beautiful sunset, you are soaking in His love. When you eat a handful of strawberries and you oooh and awee about how amazing they are, you are acknowledging God's love for you. When you choose His creations as your food, you are filling your body with God's love, life, and happiness. To eat from God's garden is to show gratitude and respect to Him. Being aware of how amazing, intricate, and unique God has made you is a vital part of deciding what to put inside your body. Choosing to eat in a manner that nourishes your body, which is both a gift and a temple of God, is a wonderful way to love God.

Sharing God's Love

The love that parents have for their children is an important aspect of nutrition. Because you love your child, you want him to thrive. As a parent, you want to see your child happy, healthy, and making the most of their potential. What you feed your child should be based on that same love. Because the food you choose for your family will either enhance your child's happiness, health, and potential, or it will harm them.

We express love to others by sharing food to them. Cooking dinner for your family is an expression of love. Surprising a friend with a care package, sharing strawberries you picked with family, and surprising a person with breakfast on their birthday are all examples of how the the need for food gives us the opportunity to share God's love.

In my studies of nutrition and reflection of the way I share food with others, I have realized that our culture has somehow arrived at a point where we often are not sharing real love with one another in the realm of food. This is because our food supply has been gradually contaminated and poisoned in the last 100 or so years with fRood. Unfortunately, it is the fRood that we pass to one another under the disguise of love. In college, whenever I came home to visit, I would make puppy chow (the chocolately, peanut buttery, sugary covered cereal) for all my little brothers. They would get so excited! After college, I got really into granola. It became a centerpiece in care packages, stockings, and birthday presents. And then my studies and research led me to a point where the truth was right before my eyes. I had fallen into the well disguised and almost genius trap set by the fRood industry. I was expressing love by giving poison to my family and friends. We have been pitched a sales campaign that advertises this fRood as love and we have been hooked, line and sinker.

Chocolate on Valentines Day, easter baskets full of candy, cookies at Christmas, candy on halloween, girl scout cookie season, and even birthday cakes are all examples of how fRood has been paired with showing love. The commercials on tv that equate giving cookies to others as love, making marshmallow crispy treats with your child, dipping cookies into milk during bonding time between father and son are examples of how the notion that we give love through giving fRood has been sold to us, at the cost of our own health and happiness.

Expressing love without fRood

When I became aware that I was harming the health of the people I loved by sharing fRood with them, I wanted to deny it. I really enjoyed making and giving treats that were appreciated and popular. It had been a surefire way to conjure up my favorite smiles on on my favorite faces. But I realized that in order to do what was right and best for those I loved, I would have to take the knowledge that I had learned and use it. I would have to find other ways to express love. Being passionate about nutrition and wanting to fill stomachs with nutrients and not poison has taken me on a journey where I have learned a great deal about love. It started with a search for new ways to express my love. Loving others requires your time and attention. It requires creativity, action, and presence. At the time, I was living in California and so I shifted my culinary focus to compiling healthy meals and snacks. A younger brother was living with me at the time and I smile every time I think of his reaction to my guacamole. He would grunt his satisfaction and praise how good it was as he dipped red peppers and celery into it. And he did this every time I made it! It never failed to make me laugh and I felt good that I was feeding him food that was nourishing and not poisonous. Instead of bringing sugary treats home when I visited, I would bring their favorite fruit. Or something new for them to try, like the passion fruit that grew in my front yard.

I also began to understand the importance of being present to each moment and the value of giving love when it is needed, as opposed to when you feel like it. The biggest realization that I came to in regards to love was this: the greatest gift of love you can give to others is your presence and attention. When your focus shifts from yourself to those around you and sharing God's love with them, the happiness and joy that you extend outwards is unparalleled. Laughter flows more freely,   you inspire and share joy, meaningful conversations happen naturally, and camaraderie is enhanced.

At that point, I also began to change my nannying style. I asked myself what my purpose was as a nanny. The answer was to help families become happier and healthier and to serve in a way that cultivated love among them. This meant focusing on activities with the children that fostered physical and mental development, happiness, and love. It meant feeding them food that fostered those same things when it was in my power. Sometimes, it meant making special meals or snacks for a mom who was trying to get healthy.

We live in a culture that makes true love difficult to express. That is especially true in regards to children, because it often means putting their best interests ahead of their wants. It is not pleasant to say no to those you love, but it is the responsibility of parents to nourish and protect their children. Their brains are not fully developed and they are not old enough to make the right decisions in many areas of their lives. It is the parent's role to teach them all they need to know in order to thrive in this life- to be happy and to discover their purpose and the plans God has for them. This often means making decisions that are not going to please your children. But you make those hard decisions because you love your children and you want what is best for them.

It is so important to understand that feeding your children based on their preferences and what they like, is not the best way to express your love. Children today gravitate towards fRood, and are not mature or knowledgeable enough to understand the importance of nutrition. As parents, it is essential that you do everything in your power to both feed them properly and teach them the hows and whys of healthy food so that they are prepared to take care of themselves when they are older.

To do this, it is necessary to break out of the pattern that advertising campaigns have created. Disassociate yourself from the cultural norm of expressing love through sweets. Think about where those habits have gotten us as a society and where they will take your children if you subscribe to that brand of nonsense. If fRood has been a way of expressing love to your children in the past, that can be changed. Although it may take some time, your family will be much closer and happier because of your decision. Brainstorm new ways to show your children affection and use your time, attention, and presence to really get to know your child, foster their spirits, and nurture their growth and development.

In the coming chapters, as I explain how fRood unravels lives, health, and happiness, it is important to remember that the solution to all the chaos it has caused lies in sight, right in God's garden.

Chapter 4
Sugarcide

" What you eat determines your state of mind and who you are." - Dr. George Watson

God created foods that were naturally sweet for our nourishment and enjoyment. Dates, bananas, and watermelon are all amazing foods with sugar that God has put on the earth. Refined sugar, though, takes the sweetness out of the package God put it into. All the vitamins, minerals, and fiber that He placed in sugar beets and sugar cane are taken out. Without the complete package, our bodies are unable to process the extracted substance efficiently. What started out as a component of nutritious and delicious food is turned into a sinister, sweet poison. For each gram of refined sugar you consume, it is 4 calories devoid of nutrients. Perhaps refined sugars should be termed shugars (shi**y sugars).

We were not created with "discretionary calories" in mind. Our bodies require a certain amount of calories each day, and to be truly healthy, all those calories need to be supplying nutrients as well. The detriment of sugar on your health does not end with empty calories though. Our bodies are simply not designed to use sugar as fuel. The results of using it as such are obesity and disease. And then you have its effects on the brain, including learning disabilities, depression, developmental problems, personality disorders, and more. Taken out its natural package containing all the vitamins, minerals, and nutrients necessary for its metabolization, sugar is forced to leach all the missing nutrients from your body. So not only are you consuming something with no nutritional value, but it also then further depletes the stores of those nutrients that you possess.

When you are nutritionally fit, your skin is radiant and soft, your eyes are bright and your hair is shiny. The nutrients in your body contribute to your beauty. To be healthy and vibrant, our bodies need to experience equilibrium. Minerals, vitamins, hormones, enzymes, and nutrients all depend on one another in order to keep your body in harmony and operating efficiently. When you are deficient in one nutrient or have one hormone that is not at the correct level, all other nutrients, hormones, and systems are thrown out of whack. Sugar upsets that delicate balance because it impacts each and every one of those areas. It leeches minerals from your bones, throws your hormones into chaos, steals vitamins in your body in order to be metabolized, and rots your insides, starting with your teeth.

Sickly Sweet

Sugar leeches calcium from your bones as well as interfering with its digestion along with magnesium. It causes chromium, copper, and phosphorus deficiencies. It depletes your body of the B vitamins, along with vitamins C and E.

Because sugar drains your body of vitamins and minerals, it impacts every facet of your health. Refined sugars specialty is nutrient deficiencies, the roots of modern day diseases.

Sugar is harmful to your brain, actually makes you less attractive, and can ruin your sex life. It causes premature aging, skin wrinkles, varicose veins, and cellulite. It causes acne, eczema, and dry skin. It contributes to all types of cancers, Alzheimer's, and causes tooth decay. It suppresses the immune system, and causes allergies to develop.

Sugar causes arthritis, osteoporosis, and inflammation. Heart shaped candy and cookies cause heart disease.

Sugar disrupts your hormone levels and endocrine organs, setting off a chain reaction that impacts your mental and physical health. It causes certain hormones to be overactive and others to be under active. Insulin, adrenalin, leptin, and sex hormones are all impacted. The human body is intricately designed and its organs, systems, and functions are all inter-dependent. When one item is out of whack, it can influence and harm the entire body.

When we consume sugar, insulin is the hormone that is secreted by the pancreas to transport the sugar from the blood into our bodies' cells. The more shugar you eat, the more insulin your pancreas must manufacture. In turn, the levels of other hormones throughout your body are impacted because of the large amount of insulin being produced.

Sugar's depletion of the B complex vitamins is especially prevalent in the case of depression and psychotic tendencies. J.I. Rodale wrote about the prevalence of low blood sugar in criminals at the time of their crime. His book, *Natural Health, Sugar, and the Criminal Mind,* is a fascinating look at the association between sugar addicts and violence. From terrible toddlers to Ivan the Terrible, the book is filled with stories about "sugar drunkards" and their violent behavior. Hitler, Napoleon, and Queen Elizabeth I were among the many examples given for sugar addicts. Hitler loved sugar so much, he would add spoonfuls of it to his wine. He ate sweet pastries constantly and always had candy near him. Is it perhaps a clue to the absolutely evil workings of his inner mind?

I found Queen Elizabeth's obsession with sugar particularly interesting. Back in 1500's, sugar was extremely hard to obtain, even with great wealth. It came only to England sporadically. Because of her love for sugar, it would make sense that she would snatch up as much as she could when these cargos arrived and gorge herself on it. And then she would be without it for a long period of time. It is worth while to note, that while Elizabeth was brilliant in politics at times, she experienced sporadic episodes of paranoia that led to executions of loyal people. During these periods of mental instability, she was indecisive and acted in direct conflict with her principles. Her behavior, which vacillated between brilliance and psychosis during her reign has stumped many historians over the years. Is it possible that sugar is the explanation?

Sneaky Sugar

Sugar is the most dangerous fRood of all. Not only is it a poison that harms our bodies, but it also is used to make other fRoods palatable. Cold cereal, pop tarts, graham crackers, and granola bars are all examples of foods that would most likely not be eaten if they didn't contain the sugars that they do. And most of those items are packed with refined white flour, hydrogenated soy oils, pesticides, and lots of other garbage that is not fit for human consumption. Chocolate milk, offered as a solution to get kids to drink their milk in order to get protein and calcium, is counter-productive, as the sugar will prevent the bodies assimilation of those nutrients. Popular "breakfast nutrition drinks" are advertised as excellent ways to give your children a healthy start to the day. Ranging between 5-7 grams of protein and 18-19 grams of sugar per serving, these drinks do not give a healthy anything to children. Vitamins or minerals they are fortified with become redundant because of the amount of sugar they add. And since sugar interferes with protein digestion, giving a child a "nutrition shake" that has 3 times the amount of sugar in it than protein, is not helpful to their health. The fact that most of the protein comes from soy is another detriment.

Sugar & Kids

Throughout my years nannying, I noticed that the more sugar kids had in their diets, the more likely they were to:

• Get sick
• Terrorize their siblings
• Forget: homework, where they put things, their chores, etc.
• Throw tantrums and talk back
• Struggle with homework
• Prefer sedentary entertainment
• Be picky eaters

The picky eater conundrum that faces so many parents is without a doubt an effect of exposing children to sugar. For as long as possible, you should avoid giving sugar to your kids. The longer they go without it, the more they will develop tastes for healthy food. While sugar is often advertised as a way to get kids to eat nutritious food, it is responsible for the kids' aversion to the taste of food in the first place. Children who control their own eating habits and therefore inhale sugary fRood, are always the children who are constantly getting sick. One child I nannied in particular, could not go two weeks without getting sick. When he was sick, he was given popsicles and sports drinks to break up the mucus and help him feel better. At a time when this child desperately needed nutrients, he was being given sugar, which just sapped his body of the nutrients that he did have and lengthened the sickness.

When children are sick, the answer is not popsicles, juice, or sugar laden "electrolyte" filled drinks. A much better choice is to make a vegetable soup out of potassium rich foods like zucchini, squash, green beans, and celery. Then puree the soup, curl up with your kid, and spoon feed them the elixir. Eliminating fRood from the diet and filling it with food will also result in kids with stronger immune systems.

Organic Doesn't Always Mean Healthy

While it is true that organic products have less pesticides and are a healthier choice than regular products, it is important to be aware that just because something is organic, does not mean that it is healthy. Organic sugar, agave syrup, maple sugar, coconut sugar, processed honey, and brown rice syrup are all still refined sugars and they will inflict damage on you just like white granulated sugar will. Perhaps a little less damage due to the fact that there is not bleach, arsenic, or additional pesticides to coat the poison, but your health and vitality will still be affected.

Buckle Up

Sugar's impact on your mental health is highly ignored. But it depletes vitamins that are vital to the functioning of your brain. The B vitamins in particular are necessary for proper mental functioning. They have such a profound impact that vitamins B1, B12, and C can be used to alleviate depression. Including sugar in your diet can also lead to a rampant disease that contributes to obesity. Not only does this disease cause your physical health to deteriorate, but it attacks your mental health, to such a degree that it is responsible for countless cases of divorce, crime, murder, and suicide. Welcome to the most dangerous roller coaster ride of all time: the blood sugar roller coaster.

Chapter 5
The Most Dangerous Roller Coaster of All Time

" If I were to name the chief cause of juvenile delinquency and of the growing crime rate, I would say it was malnutrition." -Dr. Francis Pottenger

Blood sugar is the source of energy for your body and your brain. It is the source of vigor and oomph. Thinking and running are both fueled by blood sugar. Maintaining a steady blood sugar level keeps your body and brain operating at peak condition. When your blood sugar is too high, it damages your bodies cells. When your blood sugar is too low, your body and brain do not have good access to energy. You actually experience partial starvation.

While most people have heard of diabetes and pre-diabetes, the condition that lies at the other end of the blood sugar scale is less known. While diabetes deals with hyperglycemia (high blood sugar), there is an equally dangerous condition at the other end of the spectrum known as hypoglycemia (low blood sugar).

Chronic low blood sugar is a condition in which people without diabetes experience low blood sugar on a daily basis. It often stems from a high sugar/refined carbohydrate diet. How is it possible that a diet high in sugar could cause low blood sugar? Because our bodies were not created and have not evolved to handle refined sugars and flours, eating sugar shocks the pancreas into overproducing insulin.

Insulin is a hormone produced by the pancreas that regulates the amount of sugar in the bloodstream. Insulin moves sugar from the bloodstream into the body's cells.

The reason your pancreas freaks out when large amounts of sugar hit your bloodstream is because it has not evolved to cope with refined sugar and carbohydrates. Your body is designed to metabolize whole foods that release sugar at a slower pace as they are digested. So when you drink a can of pop and all of the sudden 40 grams of sugar hit the bloodstream, your pancreas goes into overdrive. It goes into emergency mode and no longer focuses on precision. It starts producing insulin like crazy. It makes so much, that it can wipe out way more sugar from your blood then it should and you are left with low blood sugar.

Low blood sugar affects the brain first. Your brain is fueled by the sugar in the blood. But unlike other cells in your body, neurons cannot store sugar for later use. It relies on moment-to-moment blood sugar to operate. Therefore, when your blood sugar drops below normal, your brain is the first to experience an energy crisis. Without an adequate supply of fuel, your brain is starving. When your brain is starving, it is impossible to think clearly, be happy, or function efficiently. Many people crave sweets, which is the most immediate fix, but it triggers the cycle all over again, leaving your blood sugar even lower than before. Other symptoms for hypoglycemia (low blood sugar) are depression, trouble concentrating, confusion, antisocial behavior, paranoia, irritability, anxiety, memory problems, violent behavior, anger, dizziness, blurred vision, poor coordination, fainting, muscle pain, headaches, chronic fatigue, exhaustion, insomnia, and even suicidal tendencies. How is it possible that your blood sugar level could have that kind of influence you ask?

Blood sugar's impact on the state of your mind is powerful. Consider how you feel when you have not eaten all day. Are you in a bad mood? It is the same for low blood sugar, but the fact that it is due to the starvation of your brain is not obvious unless you understand the pattern that low blood sugar induces.

It is the most ignored condition in all of the United States and yet is very possibly the most prevalent disease today. As far back as 1960, doctors estimated that there were anywhere from three to ten times as many people with hypoglycemia as there were with diabetes. Of course, today with nearly 10% of the population having diabetes, those statistics would mean that at the very least, 33% of the population is hypoglycemic.

Brilliant doctors who worked in the 50's, 60's and 70's began to note the changes in our society that were linked to the increase of sugar and refined starches in the diets of the American people. They were not performing questionably authentic research in a lab. Working with patients hands on, they were able to fix a staggering amount of problems that arise from hypoglycemia: unhappy marriages, juvenile delinquency, depression, schizophrenia, poor grades, children's behavior, chronic fatigue, manic depressive psychosis, and a host of other issues. People who had been suffering for up to twenty years who had seen psychologists and all sorts of specialists were finally granted respite from their afflictions when smart doctors discovered that they were dealing with chronic low blood sugar and taught them proper nutrition.

Perhaps as you read this, you are thinking that it is slightly ridiculous and that if there was a syndrome as serious and widespread as this, then you would have heard about it from doctors, the news, or the media. I believe there are very specific reasons why the issue of low blood sugar is not publicized or being dealt with.

• Because the only way to effectively control hypoglycemia is to adopt a no refined sugar/no fast-absorbing carbohydrate diet, the fRood industry certainly does not want people to become aware of this rampant disease.

- There is no money to be made with this diagnosis in the medical world. The only effective way to fix the problem is proper nutrition. Therefore doctors would not be able to prescribe instant fix pills that we are so expectant of today. The idea that to be healthy we must actually change the habits that hurt our health in the first place is not a popular one.
- Instead, doctors often view the symptoms (depression, anxiety, adhd) as syndromes themselves and prescribe drugs to deal with those (aderol, anti-depressants, zanex). The pharmaceutical companies make money, but often times the medications worsen the situation (like when anti-depressants cause suicidal thoughts). Could it be because the medications are attempting to treat symptoms while ignoring the root cause of the symptoms?
- Because the symptoms of hypoglycemia are so varied and many, it can be difficult to diagnose. When facing any sort of disease, though, diet should always be evaluated immediately to see if there is a possibility that malnutrition brought about the problem.

Low blood sugar's high impact over time

Consider what happens when you cycle through the blood sugar roller coaster multiple times each day, every day, for years and years. All of those symptoms become so commonplace and present that they seem as though they are separate syndromes. Think of all the medication prescribed for depression, anxiety, and all the other problems that hypoglycemia can cause. Those symptoms begin to take over your life and direct your behavior and choices more and more. Sometimes, it occurs to the point where you start to think that they are simply part of your personality, when the problem is that you are starving for nutrients and being poisoned on a daily basis.

Pre-Pre-Diabetes?

If you eat a high refined sugar/carbohydrate diet, your pancreas is overworked. It has to produce a high amount of insulin for your body to handle that sugar. Type 2 Diabetes is a condition where the body does not make enough insulin. Is it possible that diets high in refined carbs wear out the pancreas to the point where it no longer functions efficiently? It seems logical. When you overwork a person or a blender, placing a greater demand on them than they are equipped to handle, they are going to crash at some point. Why would the pancreas be any different? It cannot be expected to handle a workload it wasn't designed for indefinitely. At some point, it is going to burn out.

The Lowering of children's potential

As awful as low blood sugar is for adults, it is catastrophic for children. Constant rides on the blood sugar roller coaster can hinder and alter brain development and their mental functions can become permanently impaired. Just like adults, they experience the host of symptoms previously mentioned, but without the maturity to control their reactions, misbehavior, tantrums, destructiveness, violence, cruelty, and absolute misery are added to the scenario. Learning becomes difficult. Concentrating in school and staying focused on homework becomes increasingly hard. I have nannied multiple children, who, even with my constant presence to keep them on task, homework takes hours and hours to complete. Kids shouldn't have to be stuck at a table doing homework like that. They need to be playing, moving, and interacting with their environment.

As a nanny, it is also my belief that hypoglycemia affects the development of children's personalities. This is because their energy and brain power that should be directed at creative and imaginative musings is constantly muted. All the time they spend with their blood sugar lower than normal is time lost. It adds up. I have seen so many children over the years who spend hours each day in a zombie-like funk where they have zero interest in activities around them. It is in these states, that they are most attracted to the television. It was the times that I had control over children's diets that I saw the most energy in them. Those were also the days that the children wanted to go outside and play tag, or roller blade, or go to the park instead of sit in front of the television.

The difference between children when they have low blood sugar and when they don't is night and day. They are happier, more talkative, and more active. The questions they ask show you that their minds are churning. New ideas for activities surface, senses of humor emerge, and there is a sparkle in their eyes. They are more enthusiastic, express more gratitude, and are more helpful.

Kids with low blood sugar are also much more likely to bicker. Siblings are always going to squabble here and there, but something is wrong if they are going at each other all of the time. As family, brothers and sisters should look out for and protect each other. Kids who ignore, are mean to, or make fun of their siblings at school or when they are with friends is a problem. In my years of nannying, I have seen children who possess such a sweet side, but more often than not it is the nasty side that is exhibited. As a society, we seem to have accepted that this is normal behavior for children. It isn't. Kids do not naturally have split personalities. They are simply sick from the fRood that they are being fed and their brains are starving for nutrients. When you understand that their behavior is because of what they are eating and not part of their personality, the importance of what goes into their bellies becomes very visible. When kids brains are starved, they feel like crap, and it is only logical that their behavior is going to be crappy too. They don't understand why they feel the way they do or even that it is not normal.

More often than not, both behavioral and learning problems in children are directly connected to the youngsters' diets. Is homework a daily stress-inducing event in your house? Do you deal with mega-tantrums on a consistent basis? Do you have preteens or teens who are always moody and ready to argue with you? What if I told you that changing the way your family eats would eradicate many of these problems?

Tyler was an intelligent and witty ten year old, for whom I was a live-in nanny along with his two siblings. He would throw tantrums, was a sore loser, once attacked his karate instructor (not part of the

38

lesson), and was very rude to adults. He had trouble getting along with kids at school, sports, and boy scouts, and was often very mean to his little sister and brother. On the other hand, if something negative was directed his way, he could not handle it and would go berserk. When I began working, the parents were worried because he had been gaining weight. He ate junk for breakfast, bought junk out of vending machines at school, and was constantly sneaking food. Although he was very smart, homework was a long and draining process with him. He would get mad, have meltdowns, and blame it all on someone else. He could also never remember where he put anything. Now, while I am aware that I am not painting the most charming picture, there was another side to him. There was a sweet Tyler who would stick up for his sister, read encyclopedias for sheer pleasure, smile ear to ear, and share his infectious laugh.   Tyler was simply dealing with malnourishment. Blood sugar swings led to anger over tiny things and the inability to control emotions.

Terrible Teens

As children turn into teenagers, many of these symptoms can become more pronounced. Stunted brain development can lead to teenagers who are prone to act impulsively because they have not learned to control their emotions. Spending years of their lives with low blood sugar while their brain is developing can prevent growth in maturity. They lack inhibition that would keep them from acting inappropriately. It is rather clear how violence, zero interest in or care about grades, and disrespect towards authority can be the results of poor diets and low blood sugar.

Now you have teenagers who are already emotionally unstable experiencing chronic low blood sugar. They are unable to reason things out, consider the consequences of their actions, or temper their emotions. This invariably leads to bad judgement and bad choices for many teenagers.

As teenagers become young adults the situation becomes more dire. Lack of ambition, no focus on the future, and the constant need for instant gratification are characteristics that are beginning to define an entire generation. Complacency becomes a defining characteristic.

There are no big plans, no American dream, and no desire to thrive. Violence is on a steep incline as proper nutrition is on a steep decline. Is there a connection? I would bet my life on it.

Besides the harm inflicted on each individual, what about the harm inflicted on our country as a whole? So many bright minds and incredible people will never maximize their potential, because it has been being damaged since they were toddlers. What if the mind that has the potential to perfect clean energy never fully develops because it is being stunted by sugar? The costs of malnourishment and sinister sugar are infinite.

Show Me the Sugar

Your child wakes up, has a glass of orange juice, two waffles with some syrup, and a couple of strawberries. Not a bad start right? Wrong. This meal makes your child's blood sugar skyrocket followed by a crash a couple hours later, right in the middle of class. So they stop paying attention and zone out. Lunch comes around and round two begins.

The level of sugar in children's diets is astounding and I guarantee that your child consumes more if it than you think they do. Outside of what they get at home, they get it at school, at friends houses, and they buy it themselves.

Of all the children I have nannied, it was always the children with a lot of sugar in their diet that epic temper tantrums were part of the daily routine. From 2-13 year olds, I have seen this time and time again. These poor kids are on constant swings from high to low blood sugar. It is no wonder they are so miserable and cranky. It is a product of sinister sugar.

Show me low blood sugar

My first experience dealing with low blood sugar came when I became the nanny for a family with a seven year old type one diabetic. Part of my job entailed testing her blood sugar level at various points throughout the day, counting and programing the carbohydrates she ate into her insulin pump, and monitoring her behavior for any signs of a problematic blood sugar level. Of everything that I learned about diabetes during that job, I was most fascinated by the link between behavior and blood sugar. Within weeks of working with her, I could tell when her blood sugar was low. Irritability, disobedience, dallying, and being mean were the key indicators. She would cry because of a simple request to get started on her homework, disregard instructions that she would normally happily follow, and refuse to test her blood sugar levels.

The seven year old diabetic had an older brother who would consistently threw what can only be described as mega tantrums. Screaming, crying, and sometimes even hitting me, he would wail about how unfair everything was, how no one loved him, and how much he hated (insert person whose "fault" it was for the meltdown). In the beginning, I was astounded and chalked it up to a spoiled child who had learned how to press the buttons of those around him. As time progressed, though, I really began to wonder. These tantrums would sometimes last more than an hour and they were never thrown because he wanted something. As I learned how to spot low blood sugar in his sister though, I began to notice that these epic meltdowns of his seemed to occur after really sugary snacks or a sugary breakfast. For instance, he would come home from school, drink a pop and eat cookies or ice cream, have some downtime, and then it would be homework time. I had to be there to keep him on task the entire time. He could barely concentrate and sometimes homework would stretch into hours. Then a tantrum would be induced. His sister would make one comment or his brother would make a joke, and that was it. What confused me was that his behavior indicated low blood sugar, but how could that be when he had consumed as much sugar as he had?

It was easy to understand how his sister's blood sugar could become low. If she was more active than normal or if the carbohydrates she ate were either incorrectly estimated or incorrectly programmed into the insulin pump, her blood sugar could become low. Her brother was not diabetic, though, so I did not see how it would be possible for low blood sugar to be the culprit for his behavior.

That question stumped me for months, until I became really interested in blood sugar levels because of a book I read. *Pure, White and Deadly* by John Yudkin is a book that was written in 1972 about the evils of sugar. The information about just how detrimental sugar is to health astounded me. As I continued to other books on the subject, I stumbled onto the prevalence and effects of chronic low blood sugar. As I read, the little boy's behavior suddenly made sense. It was his high sugar and refined carbohydrate intake that caused his low blood sugar.

It was around that time that I began to work for a family that consumed more sugar than I had ever seen. Their pantry was loaded with everything from poptarts, sugary cereal, donuts, candy, cookies, fruit snacks, and other things. Their freezer had ice cream, popsicles, and more candy. The refrigerator was loaded down with pop, juice, gatorade, and energy drinks. The children (13, 9, and 2.5) were allowed to eat and snack as they pleased, with all the fRood in the pantry being reachable to even the littlest arms. What amazed me most was that the entire family was thin. The two oldest children were rail thin and the mother expressed concern that the toddler had lost weight and it was a common occurrence for him to refuse to eat. I was told that anything I could get him to eat was great. A breakfast of glazed chocolate donut holes was considered a successful meal. By the time I got to work in the morning, the two older children were already on their way to school and so it was the toddler that I fed the most. The dishes from the older kids always pinpointed what they ate though. Waffles slathered in either maple or strawberry syrup (pure HFCS), or some sort of sugary cereal was the typical breakfast for these two. They didn't eat very much of it though. The toddler did not drink any water when I began working there. Juice was practically the only thing placed in his bottle. I soon began to realize that the older kids only ate fRood. They were suspicious of anything that did not come in a wrapper and home cooked meals were barely touched. This is when it got interesting.

Up until then, the children I had nannied who had severe sweet teeth tended to overeat. They would eat food, but were always hankering after for sweet snacks and desserts. The dietary pattern of these kids was different. They never overate, but they only had interest in eating fRood. I found out that the nine year old gave away her school lunch to friends and would only eat dessert.

When I picked up the older children from school, they reminded me of zombies. They would be zonked out, literally in a daze, not remembering what they did during recess or what they learned. They would grate on each others' nerves the entire ride home. Doing homework would take hours sometimes and required my constant attention. These children were not unintelligent though. They were simply trying to function on low blood sugar. After watching the habits of these kids closely, I realized that their sugar consumption ranged from 150-200 grams of sugar each day. Although these kids were thin, they were severely malnourished.

Family Life with Low Blood Sugar

If members of a family all possess hypoglycemia, think of the needless stress and negativity that is introduced into their lives. If any combination of the symptoms are present, the overall mood and atmosphere will undoubtedly be influenced. Exhausted parents, sullen teenagers, and riotous children do not compile a combination of factors that make for a happy home or healthy marriage. I simply cannot stress the importance of good nutrition for a happy home enough.

My heart goes out to mothers who work hard to do special things for their children. They often spend hours and hours putting together something special, only to have their kids' negative attitudes ruin the entire experience. What was supposed to be a fun vacation, activity, or day turns into a nightmare, and all that time and energy moms put into the event feels like a waste. It is easy to feel under appreciated in these circumstances or wonder "why bother?".

The problem is so simple. It isn't that kids simply don't care about the things that are done for them. It is that they feel badly. So they act badly. Health affects the behavior of children much more than adults because they lack the inhibitions that adults have. For instance, I might be really upset with someone, but I control my reaction because I am mature enough to weigh the consequences. A disobedient child on the other hand, doesn't have the capability to do so when he has no energy to think rationally in the first place.

In arguments among family members, sometimes things are said that cross the line. These sorts of things are often said solely to hurt the other person. Often times, they are not even truly believed. What determines whether that line is crossed? Low blood sugar can be a factor. This is because when people, especially children, feel miserable, it prompts them to treat others miserably. Misery loves company.

Maintaining control of your emotions depends on mental health, which depends on proper nutrition. We all have weak points in our character, and malnutrition will worsen those weaknesses. Whether you tend to melancholy, flying off the handle, or distraction, a diet of fRood will exaggerate the problem.

As I read old school books, I was thrilled to learn about doctors and psychologists who helped patients gain back their mental health through nutrition. I minored in psychology in college and never learned anything about nutrition's connection to mental health. To backtrack in time and discover that there were psychologists using nutrition 50 years ago to fix patient's mental problems was a revelation.

Chapter 6
fRood Addiction

*" Before you can break out of prison, you must first
realize you are locked up." Dr. Robert Anthony*

fRood Addiction:
1. The inability to eat a healthy diet due to constant cravings for fRood
   as a result of... SUGAR.

fRood addiction is the most prevalent and one of the most
dangerous addictions in our society today. Anyone in denial of the fact
that sugar is addictive need only watch children throw tantrums when
they are denied candy at the store, diabetics indulge their sweet tooth,
or teenagers that cannot put down the soda.

Being overweight can cause substantial emotional pain. No
one enjoys being confined to wheel chairs, unable to move freely, or
dealing with the self-consciousness that accompanies obesity. Women
ache to be beautiful and yearn to be thin. How is it in a society so
obsessed with outward appearances, that ⅔ of the population is
overweight?

All the research has led to this insight: That we all eat more calories than we burn and do not exercise enough. There seems to be no answer why. It has been deemed unclear, not well understood, blah blah blah. It astounds me that this is the explanation that the most "credentialed" and intelligent researchers and scientists have come up with. I believe that there is one simple truth that has been dismissed and disguised because of money: Sugar is just as addictive and harmful as substances like cocaine, caffeine, and cigarettes. What makes sugar so incredibly dangerous and threatening to health is that it is passed off to us, and to CHILDREN, as food.

The sneaking of an addictive substance into the food supply means that everyone is exposed to it from infancy. Just like some people can smoke socially, do drugs recreationally, and drink alcohol occasionally, some people can handle indulging their sweet tooth sparingly. However if you look at the health epidemic today, it is blatantly obvious that fRood addictions are just as prevalent, if not more so, than drugs, tobacco, or alcohol addiction.

There is an on going struggle between moms and kids over vegetables. This is especially true in regards to toddlers. I have seen more children between the ages of 2 and 4 who refuse to eat vegetables than I would care to see in my life. I have also noticed two characteristics about the homes that these children live in. The pantries in their houses are filled with a vast array of fRood and their parents allow them to eat the fRood at will. Of course the children are going to refuse to eat vegetables under these circumstances, because their parents' behavior has taught them that the fRood in the pantry is food. A toddler doesn't understand that he needs to eat vegetables for his health. He cannot make the distinction that fRood is quite different from food. All he knows is that fRood tastes much better than the green things on his plate, and so he will do everything in his power to be given the fRood. Toddlers should not be exposed to refined sugar. It ruins their health and is the reason they refuse to eat healthy foods. Besides the impact on their health, the impact of eating sugary froods for breakfast, snack time, lunchtime, and after dinner is that kids don't understand why they should have to eat other less appetizing foods at dinner. And many moms react to the picky eater syndrome by fearing that children aren't getting enough to eat, so they let their children eat the fRood. That choice simply worsens and prolongs the situation.

While experts today attribute the combination of diet and lifestyle to the obesity epidemic, they ignore the impact that diet has on lifestyle itself. fRood depletes energy, depresses brain activity, and induces lethargy. Eating sugar does not lead to a desire to hit the trails or play outside with your children. It leads to an exhaustion that makes you crave more sugar and makes couch time in front of the TV the most appealing activity.

Sugar is an addictive substance. It costs money, your mental and physical health, and your happiness. It causes people to eat more and move less, which is ironic considering the popular anti-obesity campaign slogan "Eat less and move more". The health crisis that is a direct result of sugar is hurting our nation now and will only snowball in the years to come.

Sugar addiction is no different from that of cigarette, alcohol, or drug addiction in the sense that it takes away your freedom and keeps you from doing the things that truly make you happy. The ways in which it differs include its accessibility, the path leading to it, and the fact that the addiction can be based on taste rather than the way it makes you feel after you ingest it.

Sugar addiction can occur outside the decision to try drugs. It is the most single accessible addiction in today's society because one must eat to live. Dealing with an addiction to sugar is also incredibly difficult because you cannot avoid it. It is at work in little bowls, at parties and friends' houses, at organic grocery stores, at sports stores, and is advertised on billboards, the radio and television. Temptation is everywhere. It is much more unlikely that coworkers put out a bowl of cigarettes to share with the office, that cocaine will be advertised during a network show's commercials, or that alcohol will be served after church on Sunday.

Whereas cigarettes are smoked and alcohol drank for the feelings that follow ingestion, fRood addiction can stem from both the feelings that follow ingestion, as well as the sensation that accompanies ingestion. A person smoking their first cigarette is unlikely to say, "Mmm I love the feeling of smoke in my lungs", but they may love the effects induced by nicotine. Someone biting into a candy bar, on the other hand, is much more likely to instantly love the taste of sugar on their tongue.

Addiction to fRood is heavily advertised in our culture. The notion that eating should be chosen based on taste departs from the logic of eating to maintain good health. But that is exactly what has occurred thanks to marketing and advertising.

There are people and institutions who declare that you cannot be addicted to food. But what is addiction really? I define it as anything that consumes your focus and keeps you from health and happiness. In other words, it is anything that prevents you from being free. You want to be able to run around and play tag with your children, but you are exhausted, that much movement would be hard, and maybe you'll just put in a movie and grab some cookies to make your kids happy. You know it's not good for little Johnny to be on the tablet all day, but if you take it away from him, you will have to entertain him yourself, and you are feeling particularly sleep deprived and cranky today and you do not want to deal with any nagging.

Think of the ways fRood prevents you from happiness. Think of the time you spend thinking about the things you want to eat. The mental struggles of staying on diets, the guilt when you stray from them, and just the fact that fRood is the thing you look forward to most in your day. These are all symptoms of addiction or withdrawal symptoms of addiction. You woke up this morning determined to walk the park, but you had a long day at work and what really sounds relaxing is a bowl of your favorite ice cream and catching up on your favorite show. You want to lose weight, but your designer coffee and pastry are the one bright spot in your morning. You would really love to get back into a sport you once loved or take up an entirely new one, but it seems like such a lost cause and you really just need some chocolate right now. You'll get started tomorrow. Does that sound familiar to you? It is a painful and frustrating cycle; it is an addiction. It is not an addiction that you wanted or that you formed by making a bad life choice, but one that still developed.

Path To Sugar Addiction

I believe there are three major roads leading to a sugar addiction. The first one is simply the taste of sugar. It is sweet and makes everything it is combined with taste amazing. The second path is the impact that sugar has on the cycle of your blood sugar. The last is the idea that sugar equals love, which has been subliminally ingrained in us thanks to marketing and advertising.

The Sweetest Addiction

Most table sugar is derived from either sugar beets or sugar cane. In their natural forms, fruits and vegetables that contain sugar are loaded with nutrients. The sweetness used to encourage healthful eating. Now, the extraction of sugar from its natural packaging encourages the opposite. Knowing that something is detrimental to your health and being unable to resist it because of how much its taste appeals to you is definitely a sign of a possible addiction. When you can't lose weight because you can't resist certain fRoods, it is because of an addiction.

The Roller Coaster You Can't Get Off

As discussed in the previous chapter, chronic low blood sugar can lead to a nasty cycle. When sugar becomes the antidote to the problem it causes, fRood addiction follows because of the constant sugar cravings. It becomes the only thing capable of lifting spirits and emotional attachments are formed.

For instance- you wake up, flood your blood with sugar (designer coffee) and feel a little better. A couple hours later though, you feel sapped and crappy. So you have a snack (granola bar) and you feel your energy pick up a bit. But by lunch time, you're tired and moody. The only thing that makes you feel a bit better is treating yourself to lunch and your favorite cookie for dessert. By the time five rolls around, you want nothing more than to curl up on the couch with some chocolate. It is an endless cycle where sugar is consumed and blood sugar soars, insulin is overproduced, and blood sugar bottoms out, leaving you feeling awful and craving sugar and starting the entire cycle again.

This pattern and cycle then begins to take over peoples lives. Chronic exhaustion, depression, lack of motivation, and lethargy overtake peoples lives all because of sugar. And although sugar is the culprit to begin with, it soon becomes the only relief, albeit temporary. Sugary fRood becomes the only thing that can be depended on lift the spirits. As the cycle becomes a permanent fixture in life, sugar becomes an addiction.

I Love You- Have a Cookie

The final path to a fRood addiction is the message we have all been conditioned with since infancy; that sugar equals love. While this idea was a brain child of marketing and advertising, we now pass along the idea from parent to child, from friend to friend, from lover to lover.

When love is expressed with sweets, the brain subconsciously links sweets and feeling love. It opens up the door to addiction. This is because when someone is sad or depressed and wants to feel better, sweets become a likely solution because they link love and happiness to sugar. And bam, all the sudden fRood can become an addiction.

Sugar becomes linked to happiness in children's minds when it is used as motivation or rewards. Because they have earned or achieved sugar, they unconsciously link sugar to those great feelings when they are proud of themselves for something. That can become a problem when they feel down in the dumps later in life and are looking for something to make them feel better.

Sugar is romanticized in our society and it happens at an extremely high cost to people we love. As children are growing, they are learning and creating the patterns for how they react to problems and emotions, which are difficult habits to break and can become lifelong struggles. The early years are critical times to ensure that your child develops healthy coping strategies for emotional pain. If children are not taught to turn to real love when facing pain or misfortune- the love of God, the love of family and friends, then they search for something else to turn to and fRood is a very convenient choice. For many children, they know they will receive it and is given "with love" by their parents. It is very easy to do without even realizing it. You want to show your child how much you love them. You want to make them happy. And they love sugar. So you express love by feeding them sugar.   Unfortunately, all the advertising companies and big food industries have poisoned and contorted the true way that love can be expressed through food.

Feeding your children whole foods, full of nutrients, vitamins, and minerals that will make your children's bodies and minds develop and thrive is the best way to show love through food. Instead we have been taught that love is expressed by making crispy rice treats with your child, sharing chocolate smooches with them, and initiating "pay it forward cookie circles". Those fRoods are harmful to your children and are not healthy expressions of love.

Kids and Sugar Addiction

fRood addiction is colossally damaging to children. Because of the fixation on their next fRood fix, they are not free to experience some of the most wonderful elements of childhood. Their minds are not free to wonder, to focus on interaction with the world around them, or to be fully engaged in the classroom. Going to the pool becomes about the concession stand. Going to a movie can't be done without candy or popcorn. The examples are endless. We have millions and millions of kids addicted to sugary fRood.   Now aside from the devastating effects it has on their development, think of what addiction itself does to the children.   It prevents them from experiencing a carefree childhood. If you have ever been addicted to something, be it alcohol, cigarettes, brownies, caffeine, or sex, you understand how your hunger for whatever the addiction is can take over your life. The consequences of addiction on children are amplified, because their development is altered by its presence.

Children who deal with sugar addictions often sneak food. In multiple situations, I have watched this cause low self-esteem, guilt, and shame in youngsters.   It is unfair that millions of children are exposed to addiction and the consequences that follow.

As children turn into adolescents, sometimes fRood can become their only source of pleasure. It is a nasty cycle where again, fRood is both the cause and solution to the problem. Although fRood is the cause of their self-consciousness and unhappiness, it is also the only thing that brings them pleasure, even if the pleasure only lasts until the ice cream container is empty.

Overcoming the fRood Addiction

Conquering an addiction to sugar can be extremely difficult for people, but it can be done. The first step is to assess how much sugar is in your diet. Unless you are so disgusted with the count that you go cold turkey, it is advisable to slowly reduce intake in steps. The first is to substitute any processed foods with ones made at home. The reason behind this is that processed foods taste horrible without sugar. When you cook treats yourself, they are fresh, and therefore do not need as much sugar to make them taste delicious. The second step is to start substituting healthier sugars in place of white sugar. Applesauce and dates can be used in baking in place of white sugar. You still get the sweetness, but you get fiber and vitamins alongside it. Agave, brown rice syrup, honey, maple syrup are still concentrated sources of sugar, and can play havoc with your blood sugar in the same manner that white sugar can.

Reducing sugar in your diet is not pain free. Common withdrawal symptoms include cravings, irritability, headaches, and even shaking. However, mother nature has provided a wide array of medicines to aid the effort. Shifting your diet to focus on vegetables and proteins will often minimize constant cravings for sweets. Within days, the haze will begin to lift, the whites of your eyes will brighten, and you will begin to experience a zest for life. You will find that as sugar disappears from your diet and healthier foods take its place, the cravings will also disappear.

But It's Not Sweets That I Overeat...

Now, you may think, 'I'm not addicted to sugar. I don't eat a ton of sweets.". That does not mean that sugar is not the reason behind your health problems and overeating. It is sugar that makes buffalo wings, pasta sauce, asian food, barbeque ribs, pizza, and deli meat taste as good as they do. If it was not for the sugar in those foods, I would be willing to bet that a lot less of them would be overeaten.

In our modern society, where we rely heavily on processed, prepared, and fast fRood, sugar seems to have a placeholder in just about everything. It is in your whole wheat bagel, your frozen dinners, your bacon, and in countless more items that you would not guess contain sugar. Sugar makes everything taste wonderful. And therein lies its connection to the present health crisis. Not only do people tend to eat more of something when it tastes good, but sugar also interferes with with the hormone that tells us when to stop eating.

The Path Back to God's Garden

The first step to reclaiming your health and your life is to acknowledge that you have a problem. Unsure whether you have an addiction to fRood? Give it up cold turkey for a week to find out. If you cruise through the weak without giving it a second thought, then I salute you and it should be easy for you to ditch fRood on a forever basis. If, however, it is a struggle, then simply admit that fRood has a hold on you.

I have found that the most successful way of breaking free from fRood is to crowd it out. Focus on the addition of healthy food and habits to your life to edge out the harmful ones. In particular, develop a ritual for when you experience a strong craving for fRood. My personal favorite is tea. Curling up on the couch with a warm cup of tea or sitting cross legged on the patio in the summer with iced tea is a game changer. It distracts from the craving and shifts your perspective, all while delivering a healthy dose of hydration and antioxidants. If tea isn't your thing, pick something else. Maybe take a walk, meditate for five minutes, eat your favorite vegetable, grab a partner and give each other a quick massage; experiment and find a habit that you enjoy that clears the craving from your mind.

Chapter 7
Digestive Distress

"There can be no such thing as good nutrition without good digestion." - Dr. Herbert Shelton

In the search for the "cure" to cancer, one does not need to look any further than the colon. Just like a sewage problem can result in disease and death if not dealt with, sewage problems in the bowel can and do lead to disease and death. The notion exists that the digestive tract is some sort of non-stick drain that rids the body of anything harmful or unneeded. That idea is far from the truth. The standard diet today breaks the laws of nature and does not respect the limitations of the body. The result is that digestive tracts have become the breeding ground for sickness and disease. The cure to diet related diseases and cancers lies in the prevention of them, and keeping the bowel clean is the first step.

The years that it seems you can get away with poor nutrition without negative effects on your health are the years that are key for prevention. A healthy lifestyle in your 20's and 30's will be reflected with health in your 50's and 60's. On the other hand, malnutrition in the 20's and 30's will be reflected in health problems later in life, if not sooner. Until we stop supporting the search for a cure by eating neon pink frosted cookies and cupcakes, we aren't going to find one.

Digestive distress is the first indication that you are using the wrong kind of fuel for your body. Chronic constipation and indigestion affect more than 63 million people in North America alone. Gas, bloating, burping, cramping, diarrhea, constipation, and heartburn are symptoms that most of us are quite familiar with.

Laxatives, ant-acids, and a plethora of other indigestion medications ease the discomfort just enough that we can continue down the taste bud pleasing path to disease. These pills come with their own retinue of side effects though. Laxatives work because they irritate the colon to the point that it spews everything out in an attempt to rid itself of the poisonous substance. The continued use of laxatives over long periods of time demolishes the elimination channel's ability to function on its own. The less efficient the bowel is, the more toxins circulate throughout the body and the more susceptible we become to disease.

We are no longer nourishing our bodies when we eat. Health has been traded for taste and convenience. It is astounding that our knowledge of how to eat has digressed to the point that it has. Indigestion is so chronic today that it is expected and accepted to be a part of life. Just because it is rampant though, does not make it normal. It only signals that we are inflicting damage on ourselves because of our dietary habits. While indigestion can stem from several factors, the four most prevalent are eating fRood, lack of fiber, cooking everything, and improperly combining food.

fRood

Humans are alive. fRood is dead. In order to thrive, you need to put living food inside your body. Besides being mostly devoid of vitamins, minerals, and fiber, fRood lacks the enzymes necessary to be properly digested. Enzymes are substances that act as catalysts to help chemical reactions take place and are essential for proper digestion. fRood is no friend to your colon either. The average American adult has anywhere from 10 to 25 pounds of thick, hardened, putrified sludge plastered to the walls of his colon. This occurs when undigested junk sticks to the mucous buildup of the colon wall and hardens to the consistency of an automobile tire. Over the years toxins pass through the colon wall and into the bloodstream, resulting in toxemia in the body. In fact, Chinese doctors have long been saying that this is the cause of disease. That mass of sludge means a smaller space for feces to pass through and also prevents nutrients from being absorbed through the colon wall.

Fiber

A healthy digestive system will eliminate the remnants of a meal no later than eighteen hours after it is consumed. The longer the time spent in its journey through the digestive tract, the more putrefaction will occur and the more difficult the final descent to the porcelain throne will be. The longer the feces spends in the colon, the more water is absorbed, which makes it compact and rocklike. Fiber is the key to speeding up bowel transit time and keeping the digestive tract clean. It increases the bulk of waste matter and provides substance for the muscles of the digestive system to act on. Without it, fecal matter putrefies, bad bacteria multiply like jack rabbits, and the conditions for disease become present.

Cook Everything!

The obsessive need to cook everything comes at a cost to health. It kills off essential enzymes present in food needed for assimilation of nutrients and kills vitamins and minerals, degrading the nutritional value of the food. While it is essential to cook certain foods for safety reasons, we should do everything in our power to eat foods raw that are safe to consume that way. Fruits, vegetables, nuts and seeds are all great examples. Roasting nuts and seeds transforms them from nutritional power houses to mediocre have-beens. No longer alive and brimming with enzymes, they are now devitalized and all the healthy fats have turned rancid. Pasteurizing milk and dairy products denatures the protein and kills the enzyme phosphatase, which is necessary for proper calcium absorption.

Improper Combining of Food

Even if you eat healthy foods, the manner in which you eat them can cause digestive difficulties. There is an obsession in our culture to eat items from every food group at every meal. These "balanced" meals that combine dairy, meat, grains, fruit, and legumes together are a pitfall of the current culture. This practice throws digestion into chaos and turns colons into cesspools.

As extraordinary as the human body is, it has limitations, that when ignored, lead to discomfort and sickness. Digestion is an extremely complicated and detail oriented process. Different types of food are digested differently. Proteins, fats, starches, and sugars are assimilated in separate ways. The location of digestion, length of time required for digestion, and enzymes required for digestion are unique to each food type. Almonds, eggs, strawberries, and brown rice are all digested differently from one another. Human digestive tracts have not evolved at the rate that fRood, restaurants, and modern methods of eating have. Stomachs, small intestines, and your colon were not designed to be bombarded with every type of food that exists at the same time, along with the poisons that comprise so much of what is considered food today. To constantly do so, prevents proper digestion and results in the breakdown of food into poisonous gases and toxins instead of nutrients.

To enjoy digestion and health as it is meant to exist, you must eat according to the laws of nature. When the bowel's limitations are respected, digestion is a smooth process. The food moves from one stage of assimilation to the next and the max amount of nutrients are absorbed by your body.

When all kinds of food are piled into the digestive tract of once, rotten things occur. First, some foods get held up in the wrong locations because they are stuck waiting for the digestion of other foods. The result is that foods rot right in your digestive tract. As the food rots, nutrients turn into toxins, some of which end up in your bloodstream.

Even if you eat a diet without added sugar, refined flours, genetically modified products, chemicals and toxins, it is very possible that you experience some form of digestive discomfort. That is because the manner in which you combine foods has an enormous impact on digestion.

Protein, starches, fats, and sugars all are processed differently, and more often than not, interfere with each other when consumed together.

- Protein digestion begins when acidic digestive juices are poured out in the stomach. Alkaline elements interfere with their digestion.
- Digestion of starches begins in the mouth with the alkaline enzyme ptyalin in the saliva and continues in the stomach. Acids halt their digestion and sugars prevent the excretion of ptyalin.
- Sugars and fruits are digested only in the intestine. When paired with proteins and starches, they prevent the secretion of digestive juices in the stomach and because they are stuck in the stomach, quickly ferment and break down into poisons that then putrefy the other food as well.
- Fats undergo digestion in the small intestine and delay the secretion of digestive juices in the stomach. When paired with proteins, they ferment and interfere with digestion. This breakdown and fermentation then putrefies the protein.

Keeping the above points in mind, it is clear that "balanced meals" create chaos in the digestive tract. When proteins and starches are eaten together, the acid and alkaline elements clash and cause indigestion. When sugars and fruits are consumed with either proteins or starches, putrefaction occurs instead of proper digestion.

Your digestive system is not a juicer that simply squeezes out whatever its needs from the items that are fed into it. The body cannot secrete multiple enzymes at the same time that act only upon their specific targets. Therefore, combining different food types ends with indigestion. It halts digestion, subjects certain food types to the wrong stomach secretions, and causes all arrays of fermentation and putrefaction to occur.

With proper digestion, starches and complex sugars are broken into simple sugars known as monosaccharides and proteins are broken down into amino-acids. Proper digestion yields nutritive materials that the body uses to maintain harmony and health in the body. When starches and sugars ferment the end results are carbon dioxide, acetic acid, and alcohol. When proteins putrefy, indol, skatol, phenol, phenyl-acetic acids, and hydrogen sulphide are the end results. The end results of putrefaction can be as poisonous as cyanide.

Looking at the various toxins listed above, symptoms of indigestion are explained. Gas, bloating, severe pain, diarrhea, heartburn, and constipation happen when food rots in our digestive tracts instead of being digested.

We also have a tendency to wash away all the digestive juices with consumption of liquids after meals. It is best to drink your water before your meals.

The Proof is in the Pudding

When I first read about food combining principles, I was intrigued. I ordered every book I could find on the subject and immediately adopted the concepts on a trial basis. The trial basis did not last for long. It had awesome effects. I noticed improvements within a week. Indigestion became a thing of the past, and I simply felt lighter and less weighed down after meals. The bottom line was that I felt energized after eating instead of wanting to take a nap. And since food is fuel, energized is how you should feel after you eat. For me, the benefits were worth the changes, and it was not long before other brave lab rats were agreeing with me.

From an ironmen to an super moms, students to executives, people who have adopted this method of food combining report back with benefits. First and foremost, their digestion disturbances disappear. Weight loss can occur as well (but certainly does not have to), because there is no snacking or mindless munching, and although there are no upper amounts set for each meal, the simplicity of the meals discourages overeating. Improved cognition, more energy, and mental clarity were also reported benefits. While it does take some time to adjust to this style, it simplifies your life and frees up brain power to concentrate on other things. Food no longer consumes your focus.

Properly combining your foods also has a long term impact on your health. Enhanced digestion means that you are getting more out of your food. Your body absorbs more vitamins and minerals and less food goes to waste. Your colon will be much cleaner as well.

While it may seem impossible to incorporate such principles into your lifestyle, it is actually quite simple in reality. The biggest hurdle is your mind because it requires a shift in the way you view food. You have to prioritize health over taste. Once you have decided to eat in a way that helps you increase your energy and feel better, proper food combining becomes a simple way to do just that.

Principles of Food Combination

- Breakfast is the time for fruit. This is because, provided you eat it on an empty stomach, fruit spends very little time in the stomach before dropping down to the small intestine, where the majority of its digestion takes place. Eating fruit by itself allows your body to absorb all the wonderful nutrients in the fruit.

- Smoothies are a great way to have fruit for breakfast. In my family smoothies are known as awesome sauce. This is because they give you an awesome start to the day, awesome energy, and awesome nutrients that help your brain function at awesome levels. Plus there is the fact that they simply taste awesome! I make one for everyone in my family each morning during smoothie season. A couple of months before I moved home to write this book, my youngest brother was out visiting me in California and I made him one each morning. Now let it be known that he "thinks" avocados are gross. He won't go near them, and yet, he declared to me each morning how good the smoothies were. Haha! I put half an avocado in his awesome sauce. This amused me to no end. It is still amusing me actually because he still doesn't know that he is getting avocado in his smoothie. Shhh.... don't tell. There have been some close calls, when he wanders into the kitchen and the evidence is in sight, but luckily, my reflexes have been like lightening. Those situations are known as code green in my house and anyone else in the kitchen at the time rushes to run interference for me. Check the recipe section out to get your dose of awesome sauce.

• If you want to incorporate protein into breakfast, you can do so by combining acidic fruits with nuts. Because of the inhibiting action of the fat, combining certain fruits with it is acceptable, because the fat prevents the fruit from fermenting before it gets to the intestines.
• Acidic fruits include berries, pineapple, sour apples, kiwi, and citrus.
• Great nuts include almonds, pecans, walnuts, hazelnuts, brazil nuts, cashews, and pistachios. Sunflower, pumpkin, and flax seeds are also good choices.

*Nuts and seeds lose a lot of nutritional value when they are roasted. Enzymes are killed and the essential fatty acids turn rancid. The best way to consume nuts is to buy them raw and soak them overnight with fresh water and a little salt. This removes the enzyme inhibitors that sometimes interfere with digestion. If you are uninterested in soaking though, raw nuts are still a better choice than anything roasted.

• Another great smoothie idea is to take your nut of choice, soak it overnight, and then use it to make a creamy smoothie. Simply blend the nuts with some water in the morning and add your fruit. Almond strawberry kiwi and pistachio raspberry are my favorites.
• This is a great breakfast for your kids before they head off to school. The combinations are full of quality protein, carbohydrates, and fatty acids that are amazing for brain development. The combinations also deliver whopping doses of vitamins, minerals, and antioxidants in an extremely digestible form. And most importantly, they will help your children avoid the steep drops in blood sugar levels that breakfasts like waffles and syrup, refined flour breakfast rolls, cereal and milk, and all the other fRood possibilities out there can cause.

• Lunch is the time for quality carbohydrates and vegetables. Because the digestion of starches begins in the mouth, fat does not inhibit its digestion, and therefore a small amount may be included.
    Some ideas:
    • Asian style brown rice stir fry with broccoli and pea pods

- Cajun spiced quinoa with bell peppers and zucchini
- Potatoes-baked or sauteed are best.
- Whole grain wraps filled with vegetables and avocado
- Sometimes, even just a hunk of dense, home made, whole-grain bread with a slice of butter and a salad.

- A snack may be essential between lunch and dinner.   This is especially true for active or growing children, athletes, and for people in professions that require activity. Some ideas:
- Guacamole and vegetables
- Peanut butter and celery
- Yogurt
- Nuts
- Salsa

- Dinner is all about protein and more vegetables. A large raw salad that is not covered in dressing should accompany the protein.

Variations of Food Combination

Food combining doesn't have to be an all or nothing extravaganza. To combine your food in this manner 100% of the time may not be doable for everyone. But there are ways to incorporate it into any lifestyle. You can prioritize. Making fruit your first meal of the day can be done by anyone. Even if it's not going to be at home, you can grab a couple of bananas or apples to go. Eating your fruit first thing in the morning does three things: Your body gets the absolute most nutrients from the fruit because there is nothing in your stomach that causes it to putrefy before it gets digested. Secondly, it stimulates your digestive and elimination tracts. Lastly, it sets a healthy tone for the day and fills your body with energy.

Some former lab rats have decided to stick with the program on an 80/20% basis. That means that 80% of the time, they combine their foods properly, and 20% of the time, they eat whatever they want to.

Other people do a during the week on/weekends off the program. Some people stick to it except for special occasions when they "go rogue". You can find what works for you and your family and do that.

There are ways to incorporate this concept without sacrificing your favorite types of food. For instance, in my family, we still have mexican night. Instead of using tortillas though, meat boats are made. Basically, romaine lettuce is piled with the meat. Instead of having beans with dinner, they were for lunch.

Asian cuisine is also a favorite in my family. Stir fried brown rice loaded with vegetables comprises lunch and then dinner is the meat and vegetable stir fry. Everyone gets to experience both parts of the cuisine, just in a way that their digestive systems appreciate.

Combining food is really about simplicity. Acknowledging the body's limitations, respecting those limitations, and nourishing the body.

Chapter 8
TV & fRood: Power Couple

" Tell me what you eat, I'll tell you who you are."
– Anthelme Brillat-Savarin

TV and fRood complement one another quite nicely when it comes to the destruction of families' health and happiness. This is because fRood takes away the energy and happiness necessary to appreciate and enjoy life and TV provides the perfect activity for a fRood fueled person while drawing people to consume even more fRood through advertisements and commercials. The epitome of the power couple's destructive force though, happens when when they are in a room together. When TV watching and fRood consumption are combined, it results in fRoodvision: a habit forming, obesity producing, happiness assassinating activity.

While it is extremely obvious that sedentary time in front of the television contributes to obesity, it is not the only problem that television poses to the health of your family. Children in particular are exposed to some very negative influence courtesy of both the shows they watch and the commercials they see.

What Television Teaches

Every time your child watches their favorite TV show, their are learning how to act. Their favorite character's attitude and behavior impact their own attitude and behavior. They are being taught morals, what's cool, and how to act by watching a character on tv. They apply what they see on tv to their own interactions with you, with friends, and with many others. Television impacts the way children view their parents. Parents are constantly portrayed in popular kid shows as unworthy of respect. Lazy, crazy, overbearing, psycho, irresponsible, and unintelligent are a few adjectives that could be used to describe various parents on those shows. TV also impacts the relationships between siblings. Often times these shows portray siblings who are always fighting, rarely expressing love to one another, and always bad mouthing each other to their friends. TV reinforces the idea in children and teenagers that it is natural, even desirable to have a lousy relationship with their parents. Keeping secrets, lying, and dealing with problems on their own are all concepts that are reinforced on these shows.

Television Causes Low Self Esteem

Television shows can fuel self consciousness in children. These shows are full of beautiful characters who are self conscious and are obsessed with the way they and others look. When children see beautiful characters who are unhappy with how they look, think about the message they receive. Not only do most children then compare themselves to these perfect looking people and often feel less attractive, but they get the message that looks are the basis of self esteem. And that is an extremely dangerous message for children to hear. I certainly would not want a child of mine or any current child that I know and love to attach their self esteem to the way they look. A child should derive his self esteem from the love that surrounds him and who he is inside.

I have seen adorable girls and awesome boys who have very serious hang ups with how they look. Hair, teeth, noses, weight, you name it, and there are kids out there who are self conscious because of these things. Seeing a beautiful nine year old girl who insists on straitening her hair after every shower because she doesn't like her natural style (awesome and gorgeous) saddens me. And although they aren't even aware of it, when other family members joke about things that children are self conscious about, they make the children even more insecure.

Television distorts reality

Television distorts the way children view food. This is because there are often characters who are portrayed consuming food in an unrealistic way. Thin girls who always seem to have food on their minds but are not active. One character in particular comes to mind. There is an episode where she is portrayed eating a tube that looks like it is about 5 pounds of fat cake filling. The message that kids get from is that your body isn't the result of the food you eat. Deciding between what is and what is not realistic is much more difficult for kids than adults when it comes to TV. Although even as adults, we often derive unrealistic opinions and beliefs based on what we see.

Let's not forget how characters on TV shows HATE vegetables because they are so gross and cartoons portray green throw up because of things like brussels sprouts. I know so many kids who automatically say "ewe I hate spinach." But when I ask if they've had it, the answer is, "well no, but I know its disgusting." They don't know that, but they have been taught that over and over and over again, courtesy of the television.

Television stunts mental development

Television comes at a cost to your child's creativity and imagination. This is because it entertains them, as opposed to them spending time learning to entertain themselves through games and play. As a kid, I spent about three hours outside almost every day. Whether it was with my brothers or friends, we created a multitude of games, all unique and intricate with rules and objectives. We would create entire towns using chalk. Everything could be turned into a game. We had different games for sledding, swimming, and jumping on the trampoline. My point is that when kids are playing they are moving and thinking and it allows their brains the opportunity to be exercised in a way that learning at school doesn't. They also learn independence, creative problem solving, and they learn how to interact with others. In front of the TV they become dependent on others for entertainment, are not faced with real life situations that stretch their minds, and watch staged interaction between others. That fake and constructed interaction still impacts the way the way your child interacts though and often times it is not for the better. That is because television is made to be funny, capture children's attention, and keep them watching. It is not designed to teach them values.

Television does not lead to happy kids

Watching television does not make children happy. They may really want to watch it, and they may like being entertained, but pay close attention to your child after the television is off. What does he have to show for his time in front of the tube? Ruddy cheeks and endorphins, which is what they get from playing outside? Are they excited and are their minds turning with questions, which is how they feel when they are in the middle of a great book? Do they feel proud of themselves and important, which is what they get from chores and being mommy's little helper? Those are not the effects that I see in children when the television gets turned off. I see children in a funk who lack energy most of the time. Think about how you feel after you are done watching TV. Is it happy, refreshed, rejuvenated? Or is it muted, dejected, with a time-to-get-back-to-reality overtone?

Time in front of the television does not qualify as quality family time. Play time with your kids is precious and should not be squandered on anything less than activities that bring families closer together, express love, and create special memories.

I am not saying that a movies cannot be incorporated into a happy family life. They should not be the norm though. An official movie night where everyone wears pajamas, snuggles on the couch, and shares a healthy snack while watching an inspirational movie is terrific. It is special if it happens on special occasions. But if time in front of the tube is your idea of spending time with your children, it is simply a cheap filler for real bonding.

The I Wants

Commercials and advertising also have huge impacts on your children. First of all, kids do not understand the concept of advertising. They do not possess the ability to differentiate between reality and marketing. When they see energetic, happy, and active kids who have just eaten sugary cereal, they don't see what adults do. That is what makes it so very dangerous to them. The advertisements they see seem real to them and why would they not? Toddlers and young children don't understand the concept of using advertising to make money. TV also gives children a case of the constant I wants because they are always being exposed to new gadgets and fRoods that look really cool. And this all begins at an extremely young age.

The most dangerous association that commercials teach your child though, has to do with love and with fRood. It teaches them to associate love with sugar. When they see parents and children dipping cookies in chocolate milk and bonding, or watch a smiling mom hug her daughter and help her stir crispy rice into sticky marshmallow, or see a chocolate company's declaration of chocolate as love, what do you think it subliminally teaches to them. It teaches them that sugar goes with love. It teaches them that sugar is how you express love. It really is an ingenious marketing tactic, but unfortunately its high cost includes the health of children.

Advertising has already succeeded in tricking most of us to express love with sugar. It has become the number one way to show affection to others. Bake them cookies. Buy her chocolates. Surprise him with his favorite desert. It has subliminally been ingrained into us.

TV distorts the purpose of food

Kids are being introduced to a food culture in which nutrition is not a priority. Popular culture, cool graphics, and sugar used to entice children to eat fRood. Spongebob yogurts, toy story fruit snacks, cartoon character graham cookies, and happy meal toys are examples of how marketing attempts to lure kids to fRood by using characters from children's shows and movies. Those are all examples of the dynamic duo of fRood and TV.

This erects an entire culture for children based on eating for pleasure. From a young age, they are presented with the idea that food should be exciting and fun. Nutrition takes a back seat. It also makes your job as a parent much harder. How are you supposed to get your child to eat their broccoli when they constantly being taught that food should be shaped like cartoon characters, neon colored, and packaged in wrapping paper?

If fRood did not have such colossally awful effects on health, I would be seriously impressed. For instance, consider football shaped candy and cookies that are right in front of the check out aisles at grocery stores. They are fun right? The packages have your favorite teams on them? How can you not get them for the party you are throwing for the game on Sunday?

fRood and TV are indeed a power couple. Together, they have the power to topple your family's health and happiness. The more TV you watch, the more fRood ads you see, and the more fRood that you eat, the more TV you will watch because you won't have the energy for anything else. Their symbiotic relationship means a downward spiral for you and an upward spiral for their profits.

Chapter 9
Food's Effect on Family Culture

"Nine-tenths of our happiness is based on health. With it, everything becomes a source of pleasure." Arthur Schopenhaurer

Having a happy family hinges on the ability to enjoy day to day life together. Enjoying your family should not be reserved for vacations; it should happen each day. Food (and fRood) have a tremendous impact on family culture. Creating a happy family environment begins with creating healthy environments within the bodies of your family. When harmony is in our bodies, minds, and spirits, we are able to live in harmony with those around us. Nourishment not only provides mental and physical well-being for the individual , but for the family as well. When each person feels good, it has a beneficial impact on others around them.

If you are tired and irritable while playing cards with your kids, teaching your daughter how to properly fold laundry, or showing your son how to wash vegetables, there is not going to be any laughter, joy, or bonding taking place. An opportunity to make your family happier just passed. Your child is only going to want to play with you if there is joy in the play. When it comes to spending time with their parents, smiles and laughter are what children are after. I have seen it time and time again. It is your love and your attention that they crave. Giving your attention to them makes them so much happier and healthier than anything you could ever buy for them.

The importance of eating together as a family cannot be overstated. Eating as a family provides nourishment for body and soul. The camaraderie, traditions, and unity that evolve at the table are priceless. Meal time is an opportunity to gather together as a family and truly love one another; to share the stories, hopes, struggles, and goals for the day. To support one another, offering unconditional love and uniting in gratitude for the blessings God has given. Food can be a wonderful catalyst to bring families closer together, but it does not automatically happen just because everyone is sitting at the same table. Family culture is cultivated each day, by the effort that parents bring to the table.

Eating with your family also takes the focus off the food itself. Kids are a lot more likely to eat their vegetables if they caught up in a lively conversation than if their only focus is how much they don't like broccoli. Some of my fondest memories as a child involve my family gathered around the kitchen table. But it is not the food (although that was also awesome) that makes the memories so special. Sunday breakfasts after church that fueled the fun activities of the day. The celebrations, reflections, and life lessons that were learned and shared at mealtimes were many, and still are, when we are gathered together.

GMF's

To create a loving and happy atmosphere, you need patience, energy, a positive attitude, and clear communication. These make life flow more smoothly. And they are ridiculously hard to have when you are fueling yourself with fRood.

When you eat fRood, you're going to have a bad 'tude.

It is practically impossible to create a positive atmosphere in your home when you have a negative atmosphere in your mind. To have fun with your kids, enjoy your kids, and be a good parent to your kids, you need to be in a good mood.

That is where good mood food (GMF) comes in. Foods filled with nutrients that furnish lasting energy for your entire self, from your mind to your muscles. Some of the favorite GMF's in my family are walnuts, home made chocolate almond milk, awesome orbs (see recipe section), and home made salsa. Packed with happiness-enhancing nutrients like vitamin c, omega 3 fatty acids, flavonoids, and caffeic acid, these foods bring people together as they eat them and as they enjoy the atmosphere fostered by GMFs' effect on the family.

Family Relationships

The example you set for your kids and the attitudes you display have more influence than you can possibly imagine.

When your kids look up to you, you have a ton of power over their tastes and preferences. Your kids learn from the example you set and will like things because you like things and dislike things simply because you dislike things. This is especially relevant in the realm of nutrition. Consider the following two scenarios.

The mayo face

Ask any of my siblings, myself included, their thoughts on mayonnaise, ranch, sour cream, or anything else in the realm of "white stuff". A painstaking grimace, followed by a request to stop making them feel like they are going to throw up is the most likely response. If you were to ask them if they ever had it though, you would receive a measured glance and then a righteous, "No, and I never will." Now, for eight people to dislike something that much that most of them have never even tasted, one might think we all witnessed some sort of traumatic event that involved white condiments. Not exactly. Growing up, we ate our salads without dressing, our sandwiches dry, and our tacos plain. But it was my dad's expression of disgust when "white stuff" was mentioned or present at family parties that the credit belongs to. I can still picture his anti-mayonnaise face, and although it makes my stomach uneasy, it also cracks me up that my dad's distaste for white colored condiments is responsible for a whole brood of white condiment despisers.

The brussels sprout face

I was attempting to get some kids that I nannied to eat more vegetables and was going through the "How do you feel about x vegetable", when I got to brussels sprouts. A flurry of "Eww gross" and "That's the most disgusting vegetable ever" came at me. When I asked if they had ever tried it, the response was "No, but my dad has and he said they taste really bad."

I rest my case. Influencing your children is not nuclear physics. They simply watch and learn. Whatever values, morals, and habits you want them to possess must be displayed by you on a daily basis.

I got such a kick out of one girl in particular that I nannied. Although she ate a junk diet when I started working for her family, she watched me and the way I ate, and it wasn't too long before her curiosity got the best of her. She was willing to try everything I brought at least once... she actually tried dried seaweed three times. Finally, after she had spat it out for the third time, I asked her why she kept wanting to try it if she thought it tasted that awful. She looked up at me and replied, "Because I want to be like you." This cool little lady reinforced the fact that adults are in a position to influence youngsters. They watch you and learn values based on what they see. The happier you are and the more loving you are, the more that they will want to be just like you. As a parent, you are the most important role model in your child's life. No one else has the scope of influence that you do. Since you love them and want them to thrive, you have to use your position of influence to teach them everything they need to know to maximize their potential.

These characteristics of happy, close-knit families don't just happen. Your children don't simply grow up and become friends with you. It is a process that starts all the way back in childhood.

Family is a sacred institution where God's love is meant through flow freely and strongly, uniting it's members and offering refuge and safety from the outside world. And yet, families are falling apart by the thousands. Divorce is rampant. And the effects that divorce has on children is unmeasurable. It will continue to impact them throughout their entire lives.

Rewarding your kids

Kids love to have fun and there is no limit to the amount of fun kids can have. As a nanny, I have worked in some interesting situations where I have been expected to achieve results (homework, clean rooms, ect) with kids who had zero consequences for lack of obedience. The question became how. The answer was to make those activities fun by bringing energy, optimism, and laughter to the table. And by giving rewards for good behavior. Water balloon fights, giving underdogs while they were swinging, and time spent focused on their favorite activity are some examples.

Food and television are not good reward systems for kids. Food should be fuel for living and fuel for children's fun. It should not be looked at as the source of fun. The worst reward system that exists is giving sweets to kids for eating their vegetables. It sends the message that sweets can be a daily habit. Giving time in front of the television as a reward sends the message that television is best way to relax and the best way to spend time after being productive. That programming will become part of your child's life. TV will become their stress relief in college and after work. The problem though, is that sitting in front of a television for hours isn't a good relaxation choice. Because it doesn't rejuvenate, nourish, or make a person happy. In contrast, it is tuning out of reality and leaves the viewer slightly depressed when he must return to reality.

Rewarding your child for good behavior by spending quality time with them doing things they love is the most awesome kind of reward they can get. Nothing can compare to giving your child an energetic you, ready to play, laugh and love them.

The Atmosphere of the Home

One of the biggest realizations that I have made in my years of nannying, as well as my own life, is that the woman of the house sets the atmosphere. We either set a tone that invites, inspires, and nourishes, or one that is unwelcoming and uninspiring. One that either draws others closer or chases them away. Think about where your children spend most of their time when they are at home and how often they seek out your company. This is very indicative of the overall atmosphere of your home.

I had been nannying for a family for about a month when I received one of my very favorite compliments. There was a thirteen year old boy in the house who loved video games and spent every moment of his free time playing them when I started working there. As the weeks passed, though, he gradually joined in activities with the rest of us. He would come outside, play ping pong, and hang out in the family room after dinner. One night when I was talking to the mom about how everything was going, she remarked that she had seen such a positive change in her son. "He spends less time in his room, is nicer to his siblings, and is much happier than he was before, and I think that is because of you." That is the kind of feedback that really made my job rewarding. Creating an atmosphere where kids got to be kids was one the best aspects of my job. All it took to get Liam out of his room was some laughter and showing him that his company was enjoyed. Kids desperately need the validation from those who care for them that they belong and that they are enjoyed.

When I decided I wanted to write this book, I moved from San Diego back to my home in Ohio where I live with my dad and four of my brothers. Since I am the only girl in the house, and since I love nutrition and cooking, it follows that I spend a decent amount of time in the kitchen. My youngest brother tries to "send me to the kitchen" when my singing and dance moves fail to impress him. I always laugh because I love the kitchen. He then gets flustered and says its a bummer that woman jokes don't bother me. I tell him I could pretend to be bothered.

It is when I'm in the kitchen, listening to music, with a pep in my step and a smile on my face as I whip up snacks or meals, that my family tends to wander in. First they ask what I'm making and then they tell me about their day. We joke and laugh and they wonder when the food will be ready to devour. The early mornings are my very favorite. Sometimes at 6:15 in the morning, I'll be making smoothies and one wise crack leads to a spontaneous ab workout courtesy of contagious laughter. That is what I call a productive start to the day.

The point is that food and a positive attitude do wonders to bring your family together. But the woman of the house is the one who sets the initial atmosphere. Are you peaceful and loving, making others want to linger and be around you, or are you rushed and stressed, making others want to stay out of your way. Men and kids respond to the atmosphere that is created by the woman of the house.

Nutrition plays a direct role in the atmosphere of the home because it determines your overall sense of well being, as well as that of your children. Each member's health impacts the relationships they have with those around them. If you have a teenage daughter who lacks energy, has low self-esteem, and is generally irritable, it is not very likely that she is going to get along with her hyperactive younger brother. Feeding your family a wholesome diet sets the atmosphere that allows you to create the close knit family you desire.

So often I hear the dismissal from parents, "Well he's a teenager". It is viewed as normal in our society for parents and teenagers to have strained relationships. This is such a shame, because children especially need their parents in those years.

What I have seen in many families is that parents have lost the ability to connect with their children. They use things like TV, feeding their children based on their preferences, and buying them stuff to connect with them. These connections, aside from not being healthy, are not meaningful, and are not lasting.

What I would like to suggest is a lifestyle full of activities that will not only make your family happier and healthier, but will help you form a connection with your children that lasts.

In every family I have worked for, it has always been clear to me how much the parents love their children. They want them to succeed, to thrive, and to be happy. What I sometimes saw, though, was that love get caught in translation. A huge gap between wanting what is best for your child and doing what is best for your child.

In my experience as a nanny, and also my experience in my own family, is that children want your attention and they want you to enjoy them. After a long day at work, parents get home and they are so exhausted that they can't muster up the energy to interact the way they really want to with their children.

Nutrition can help that, and I can attest from personal experience, that this is the kind of interaction with your kids that is going to keep you close through those teenage years and also as adults. Many people between the ages of 25 and 30 go home, or have their parents come visit because they feel obligated. Not because they enjoy it. But shouldn't joy be part of seeing your family. When I lived in California and would come home to visit, I was stoked. I would literally count down the days because I love spending time with my family. I enjoy the fun shenanigans and getting whopped on in ping pong by my younger brothers. I enjoy great conversations with my dad, poker night, and watching my younger brothers play soccer. My brothers will wrestle, and I will invariably get put in a headlock, but will make a great escape using my only weapon- tickling. I always know that we will laugh. I have one younger brother in particular, whose laugh is contagious. If he starts, you start, end of story. If it is summer time and we are lucky enough to get a great thunderstorm, I know that all my brothers will be ready to tear through the yard and possibly do a rain dance. I will cook food and they will all eat it and make some joke about women in the kitchen, after which they will do all the dishes.

This environment didn't just happen one day. My family did not grow up and decide one day that we were going to be close. It was cultivated and is still being cultivated each day.

Time spent watching tv and playing video games creates the illusion of bonding, but there is really no quality interaction taking place. The focus is not on either of you. It is on the screen. If you want to make your family strong and loving, you need to devote two things to your goal. Your time and your attention. You don't have to spend money. It could be playing catch outside. It could be dancing around the kitchen twirling your daughter and telling her how beautiful she is. That is what your children want and that is what they need.

As you undertake this journey into health it is important to keep in mind the most important nutrient of all: love. It is the reason that you starting down the path. It is because you love your family and you want them to thrive. Love has to be the theme. It is the only way that you can accomplish the transition from fRood to food. Sitting down with your children at dinner and eating that broccoli with them, smiling and explaining that the broccoli is going to help them become big and strong like their dad is going to yield much more positive results than simply dishing it out and commanding that it be eaten.

Make sure that you tell your children that you are making this change because you love them. When you incorporate love, laughter, and attention, you will be amazed at what you can achieve with your children. Because those are the nutrients they need the most from you, that only you can provide. And they will respond to it. It might take some time and and there are going to be bumps in the road, but love will prevail. Children want to be the center of your attention and know that you love them. And when you provide, they will surprise you. I know they surprise me and I am not even a parent. When you provide nutrition of the soul to children, they will recapture your heart day after day.

Chapter 10
Pure Play

" We are never more fully alive, more completely ourselves, or more deeply engrossed in anything than when we are playing" Charles Schaefer

The art of play, in its most pure and simple form is disappearing from our world. Edged out by mindless entertainment and overly structured activities, it is an endangered recreation that fewer and fewer get to experience. While its extinction is a debilitating blow to families as a whole, it's most dramatic impact is on children. Lack of play comes at a substantial cost to their physical, mental, and spiritual development.

Whether a person is 8, 16, 29, or 55, the need for pure play is a vital necessity in life. It satisfies a desire deep within, connecting us to those with whom we play, to the world in which we live, and to the spirit of life. The ability to be yourself, move spontaneously, and be wild, is nourishment to our minds, bodies, and souls. The need for play transcends age, occupation, and personality.

Pure play is any activity lacking structure that includes movement and imagination.

Consider the following scenarios.

Scenario 1

A dad takes his family on vacation to Nantucket. One day, they head to the beach. His kids play in the waves for awhile while he sits in the sand. 15 minutes later, his 10 year old son comes running up and asks him to come in the water too. He responds no. The son starts to beg. "Please dad, just come out partly into the water. You don't even have to go in above your knees. Please!" "No, I've got shoes on", is the response. The begging continues for about 10 minutes and ends with the dad getting annoyed and telling his kid to stop bothering him. Dejected, the boy finally shuffles away to rejoin his siblings.

Scenario 2

A dad takes his family on vacation to a beach in South Carolina. One day, he gets an air mattress and blows it up, loads it with his kids, and hauls it out into the waves. With the waves thrashing it around, all the kids are attempting to stand up and surf on the mattress. They are holding hands, trying to help each other balance, and getting tossed off left and right. The dad is right there keeping his eyes on all of them, laughing with them as they fall, and keeping the mattress from being swept back to the beach. None of the kids are in the least bit scared or worried. They can simply be wild, laugh, and have the time of their lives because they know they are safe. An hour later, they all lie on the beach, exhausted and all smiles, as other kids congregate around them, wondering if they can join in the fun.

The stark contrast between the two fathers boils down to a single factor. While the first dad is passively watching his kids, the second dad is actively playing with his kids. The memory of the first kids will either not include their dad or it will be that he wouldn't play with them. The second group of children now have a lifelong memory that revolves around their dad.

Both fathers' actions are determining both the present and future relationships he has with his kids, but the outcomes will be much different. There is a connection between the relationship parents have with their children when they are kids and the one they will have when the kids are adults. It is when they are young, that the foundation and tone of the relationship for years to come is laid. Will it be one of enjoyment and deep connection?

In all seriousness, play lays the right foundation for establishing strong bonds between parents and children that will extend through decades.

The Family that Plays Together

When parents play with their children, there are a few extremely important things that occur without effort.

Firstly, they learn to enjoy each other. The quality of laughter, joy, and jokes that arise in play are exclusive to play. This enjoyment makes parenthood fulfilling and boosts children's self esteem because they are receiving an assurance that they desperately need: the knowledge that their parents (the most important people in their orbit) enjoy their company and are delighted to spend time with them. That mutual enjoyment extends throughout the years, from childhood through the teenage years and into adulthood. Not only does it nurture your relationship now, but it also builds and strengthens it for the future. It sets the stage for a lifelong bond with your children that results their visiting and spending time with you as adults because they genuinely enjoy you and not because of a sense of familial obligation.

Secondly, parents and children learn about one another through play. Play allows us the chance to be the most true versions of ourselves. The version that God loved the idea of so much, He went ahead and created. When one plays, insecurities, worries, and pretenses fall away, revealing who that person really is. Differences and similarities emerge and are celebrated. The better family members know one another, the stronger and deeper their connection can grow over the years. For parents, playing with your children teaches you how to communicate with them. It helps you to better understand them, gives you a peak inside their world, and gives you the opportunity to guide them. For children, playing with their parents gives them a chance to experience their parents as people. Much of the time, parental roles and responsibilities make it difficult for parents to share their personalities with their kids. Taking time to play lets kids experience you intimately while your concentration is only on having fun with them.

Thirdly, playing helps develop the most natural and true bond that parents can have with children because there is no buffer between the interaction. You are not reacting to outside stimuli like when you "bond" over a movie. It is just you and your family. Each person's unique personality contributes to an atmosphere of fun, of belonging, and of love. The feeling of belonging that emerges in play is of the utmost importance for children. It you look at most teens and preteens today, it is not difficult to see that they are searching for that exact feeling. Everyone wants to belong. If kids feel that sense of belonging with their family, though, they do not have to go to such extremes to find it elsewhere. It is less likely that they will turn to sex, drugs, or alcohol in the hopes of belonging.

No Time for Play

I have noticed over the years that kids tend to spend their free time in two ways: immersed in mindless entertainment (technology) or engaged in structured recreation (sports, activities with set rules and procedures). The problem is that their lives are devoid of an extremely important element. PLAY.

While I am not arguing the benefits of structured recreation for kids, I do think that it is critical that it be balanced with pure play. Particularly for younger children.

If your child is at school from 8-3, comes home does homework, has soccer practice or a piano lesson, and then spends a couple hours watching tv or playing video games, that's not a bad day right? They were active, got their school work done, and then got to relax and hang out for a bit. That conclusion is too simple, and my experience as a nanny has shown me that it is inaccurate.

Parents are sometimes adamant that homework be done first thing when children get home from school. While I understand that is preferred to get it done so that it doesn't become an issue later (at bedtime or the morning before school) I always felt terrible leading kids through this routine. Here's why.

When kids get out of school, they have spent the better part of the day confined to a desk with their brains being inundated with information. Besides a short recess and gym class if they are lucky, they have been given zero opportunity to tap into their energy reserves. Between malnutrition and the fact that most kids don't have a proper outlet for expending their energy, it is no wonder why so many kids deal with ADD, ADHD, and hyperactivity. We've taken beings loaded with energy who are meant to be playing and confined them to hours and hours of stillness. This is particularly relevant for boys. Maybe the syndromes and learning problems that abound today occur partly because children are placed into an atmosphere that is contrary to nature.

I was extremely fortunate to be home schooled for most of my years until high school and my day went something like this. After breakfast and morning prayers, school started. Typically this was about 8 in the morning. We all had our lesson plans and knew that as soon as our school work was done for the day, we were free. 80% of the time, the school day was over for me by noon. Lunch time was followed by recess outside, which typically lasted 3 to 4 hours, before it was time to come in for chores, go to activities, have dinner, showers, night prayers and go to bed. Bedtime was usually between 7 and 8 o'clock. There were never any arguments or tantrums related to bedtime though. We were all so tired that we gladly crawled into bed and closed our eyes. We were all played out.

Pure Play and Children's Development

With today's tendency to focus so intensely on children's performance in school, sports, and other activities, the importance of play is often overlooked. The concept that has been popularized is that children must partake in "learning activities" and "structured recreation" in order for the mind to develop. What true play offers though, is unattainable through other activities.

Pure play exercises the brain. When they are no rules and no set courses of action, the brain is constantly stimulated by the situations, atmospheres, and people encountered. Pure play will never reproduce the same moment, the same experience. Each session of play will evolve into something entirely its own. It is in that evolution and change that the brain develops phenomenally.

Pure play helps children to learn about themselves, become confident in themselves, and grow in their identity. Because play allows children to be the truest forms of themselves, it is in play where they have the capacity to truly grow into the people God created them to be.

Pure play fosters socialization. When children play with others, they learn how to interact with others naturally and comfortably. They learn essential skills of getting along with others, resolving disputes, and the importance of teamwork in life.

Pure play teaches creative problem solving. Exposure to new and constantly changing situations is practice for children to evolve and deal with changes in their lives. When there are no rules that confine or limit thought processes, anything is possible. It is that circumstance that allows children to learn different approaches for dealing with conflict and cultivates thinking outside of the status quo.

Pure play results in laughter and stories that become special memories. Play sets the stage for comedy. Whether its wipeouts, or inside jokes that will continued to be laughed at for years to come, laughter follows play.

When Play occurs outside, it allows children to learn about life by experiencing nature. It also instills a wonder, respect, and gratitude for our world. Limitations and possibilities are learned first hand. Experiencing things hands on is a much better way to learn than out of a book or from a teacher.

Ultimately, playing is practice for life. Kids develop and sharpen skills they need later in life. The fact that it happens naturally, with no lesson planning needed is truly incredible. There is such a tendency to make everything technical and complicated today. It is in simplicity that the things that matter most will thrive.

Play's impact on Nutrition

Just as nutrition influences all other aspects of your life, it also affects play. In fact, play is possibly the most awesome tool to improve your family's health. Besides the fact that it gets people off the couch and moving, play can be a huge motivator for children to eat healthy.

As a nanny, I was committed to doing everything in my power to foster the development of the children in my care. For me, that meant allowing children to spend time in front of the television as little as possible. I also didn't want to be a strict dictator whose favorite word was no. Over the years, I perfected the art of subtle misdirection. When I first started nannying kids who were used to spending free time with technology, I would tell them that they could have half an hour to play video games or watch tv after we spent some time outside. When we went out, I didn't just park myself in a chair and tell them to play. I initiated the experience. Whether I ran around chasing them, put on rollerblades and helped choreograph "olympic performances", pretended I was in the army, or rolled around in the dirt, I played with them. And here is what happened. They forgot about wanting to go inside to watch tv. They wanted to stay outside longer. As soon as I picked up children from school, their first question was, "Can we go outside when we get home?" How awesome is that? But it gets even better.

I soon realized that playing with kids put me in a position of power. They wanted to get out there so badly, that they would volunteer to help with various chores to get out there sooner. I took it one step further. I brought nutrition into it. I started incorporating healthy foods into snack time with the explanation that if they wanted to have the energy to play, they needed to eat healthy food. I would hint at all the fun we were going to have and display how excited I was to get out there. Result? They would scarf that food down. This worked on toddlers to teenagers.

Playmates

Playtime may seem like its out of the question for you because of time constraints. Make some sacrifices if you have to. Give up your gym membership and chase your kids around the yard (cardio) and swing them into the air (weightlifting). I knew a dad who used to make his twelve year old walk on the treadmill for half an hour each day. The dad spent time in the gym each day as well. I often wanted to ask him why he didn't just take his boy outside and kick around a soccer ball or throw a football with him.

Besides finding time to play with your kids, it is important to find good playmates for them. Join up with friends who have kids around the same age as you and take turns hosting play dates. Not only does that give each parent some free time to get stuff done, but the kids learn how to entertain themselves and socialize. Some of my favorite memories from childhood involve games played when families from our church congregated together. Epic games of kick the can, red rover, capture the flag, spud, dodgeball, and tennis ball wars fostered friendships, a love of play, and an early bedtime. Build yourself a community of friends that share the same values as you and are just as dedicated as you are to achieving health for their families.

What are you waiting for? Get out there and play!

Chapter 11
Erotic Eating

" *One cannot think well, love well, sleep well, if one has not dined well.*"
-Virginia Woolf

A friend of mine used to open up abstinence speeches to teens with the question, "Who wants to learn how to have amazing sex?" Inevitably, every hand in the room would raise. Why? Because we are sexual beings and that yearning for sexual satiety is an almost universal desire. While there are many factors that influence sexuality, nutrition is one of the most overlooked and important components of a healthy sexuality.

Sexuality and food are intimately related, but it is the relationship that matters least that is the focus of today's culture. Food's ability to aid in seduction is well known, but the influence it has on the quality of sex itself is mostly ignored.

Using food to seduce the object of our affection is a timeless tradition. I'll bet even cave men used delicacies they gathered to start fires in the bedrock. Nowadays, chocolate seems to be ultimate weapon of seduction on the menu. Second only to alcohol. The concept is counter operative though, because the only capability chocolate has in the bedroom is to diminish the sexual experience.

How then has chocolate come to be such a widely accepted expression of romantic love? Why is it at the center of Valentine's Day and considered an aphrodisiac? Is it because since the dawn of time man has noticed that when he brings truffles home to his wife he gets lucky? Or is it because marketing has simply implanted that idea into our minds?

It is the deeper connection that food has to sex- its impact on the body and on the organs responsible for sexuality- that is the most powerful. It is this connection that influences the sexual drive, sexual experience, and sexual satisfaction. A romantic, candle lit dinner may grant you access to sex, but it is the healthy, nutrient packed meal that will grant you access to super sex (note: this is not an instant fix. It takes many nutritious meals.).

Instead of using fRood that delivers pleasure only to your taste buds to instigate good vibrations, it is much better to use food that is going to enhance pleasure during lovemaking. Seduction by raspberries? Yes please.

If that notion seems ridiculous, take a moment and consider the reason behind your reaction. Perhaps it is because today we are more likely to be seduced by fRood than another person.

Someone once told me that prepared food was somewhat seductive. "Think about it," he told me, "a prepared recipe, with great flavor and great presentation really puts my body in the mood to eat a lot, probably even drool a little if it really looks and smells good." I laughed at that and realized that I needed to figure out how to make people drool over almonds. While it began as a joke, the idea of food and seduction kept coming back to mind.

The word seduction conjures up the image of a sensual person luring another into bed. Their oozing sex appeal makes it impossible to say no. How often is that image reality though? I would argue that there is a much more common seduction that takes place. Today, we watch a beautiful woman deep within the throws of a chocolate-gasm in a commercial and then run to the store to buy that fRood. The advertisement uses sensuality to seduce the consumer into bed with fRood.

Watching chocolate-gasms in commercials irks me. This is because eating all that fRood and chocolate that you are lured to buy because of its association to steamy sex can actually prevent you from having steamy sex. fRood destroys your vitality, can shut down the hormones responsible for your sex drive, and drains your bodies of the vitamins and minerals necessary for a healthy sex drive.

You must decide which form of seduction you want in your life. Do you want to be seduced by fRood, or do you want to possess the vibrancy, vitality, and virility to be the seducer?

Sex Problems?

It is ironic that in our sex crazed nation, "sexual problems" are at an all time high. Men have problems with erectile dysfunction and premature ejaculation. Women suffer from the lack of arousal, lubrication, and orgasm. Both suffer from lack of libido and fertility issues. These problems often lead to self-doubt, self-consciousness, and problems in relationships. It leads to men questioning their manhoods and women wondering what is wrong with themselves. Much of the time, however, these problems are rooted in nutrition. What appears to be a sex problem is actually a malnutrition issue. If a person is experiencing trouble in the bedroom, it is likely that other aspects of their health are suffering as well. Erectile disfunction is actually one of the first signs that a man's cardiovascular health is in jeopardy. The proper remedy is to treat the root problem, not the symptom.

One of the most important foundations for a steamy sex life is nutrition. Every calorie needed by your body is a calorie that you can choose to consume in one of two ways. It can be a calorie that will enhance your energy, health, and sex life, or a calorie that diminishes those things. The choice belongs to you.

Sexy Nutrition

Dr. Bernard Jensen noted in his book *Love, Sex, and Nutrition*, that throughout the fifty-five years of his practice, it was the married couples with active sex lives that were the healthiest of his patients. Just as health impacts sex, the opposite is true. Sex improves blood circulation, revitalizes the glands, and strengthens the immune system.

Sexual satisfaction hinges on the body's ability to catalyze all the conditions necessary for the sexual experience to culminate in a climax. First and foremost, the body needs energy to fuel sex. When the body is exhausted, stressed, or unwell, desire for sex is diminished. The body needs rest and proper nourishment in order for us to have a healthy sexual appetite. As Dr. Paavo Airola put it in *Sex & Nutrition*, "Sexual energy is sparked by excess energy." In addition to stamina, a vibrant and satisfying sex life requires good blood circulation, proper endocrine gland function, and a well-nourished brain.

When arousal occurs, blood flow to the genitals increases. This blood flow results in erections in men and an increase in clitoral size for women. Proper blood flow also influences the most powerful sexual organ in the body, the brain. Poor blood flow disrupts the hormone signals that travel back and forth between the brain and genitals. Those signals are crucial for the climb to the peak of the sexual experience. Without them, it is likely that one will get caught in sexual limbo. Initial arousal may be experienced, but chemicals and secretions essential to propel the body towards climax may be lost in translation without proper blood flow.

The endocrine system is made up of glands throughout the body that produce hormones. While only some of the glands produce sex hormones, they all impact the sex life because the endocrine glands are interdependent. When one gland is under active or weak, it stresses the others, and lowers overall health. It is the sex hormones that stimulate sexual excitement and produce the feel good chemicals in the body that make sex so pleasurable. Doses of testosterone, phenylethylamine, LHRH, adrenalin, and oxytocin at various intervals of intertwinement help the body climb towards the pinnacle. Without all the wonderful secretions, a person is more likely to lose themselves in planning dinner than in throws of passion.

The most important sexual organ, the brain is where desire originates. It is where an emotional response to another person leads to arousal. It is where the sensations experienced in an intimate dance are translated to sexual excitement. For sexual stimulation to occur though, the brain must be firing on all pistons and must have access to mojo. Since we know the negative effects that fRood has on the body, it is easy to understand how a fRood filled diet destroys the ability to have a vibrant sex life.

The effects of fRood on sexuality compound as you age. What you were able to get away with in your 20's is not going to be the same in your 30's 40's, or 50's. Lasting sexual satisfaction relies on continued attention to nutrition.

Men who claim that salads are for women and pride themselves on being carnivorous, manly men, miss out on the nutrients that they need to be virile men. It is the men who make room in their diets for plants and know that salads are the key to enjoying and pleasing their women that ooze virility.

Women under the impression that orgasms rely solely on the bedroom skills of their men need to acknowledge nutrition's impact on their sexual experience. Before the man's finesse between the sheets becomes suspect in the case of the missing O, a woman needs to examine her diet and super charge it for sex.

When a loving couple has endocrine glands that are in peak condition, good blood flows, and nourished brains, it is a situation ripe for sexual delight. A seductive look, word, or touch enkindles emotion, triggers the glands, and activates the nervous system. The heart begins to race, tissues swell with blood, adrenalin is released, and the sex glands secrete hormones. As arousal deepens, every touch fires off nerve impulses that travel to the brain, triggering the release of endorphins and pleasure-producing chemicals. The collision of senses, sensitized nerve endings, and intimate contact ignite sexual excitement. As the body's signals to the mind intensify, the pleasure center in the brain takes control. Oxytocin is released, initiating the involuntary tremors that accompany orgasm.

Sex and Healthy Homes

Having a good sex life in marriage is an important component of the home atmosphere. Sexuality (or lack thereof) affects other aspects of marriage, which affects the family as a whole. Sex strengthens a married couple's bond and keeps them in tune with one another. As the knowledgeable Dr. Bernard Jensen states in his book, *Love, Sex, & Nutrition,* "Sex is the body's version of love". It is meant to be a source of joy, a means of communication, and an intimate connection full of pleasure in marriage. Uniting bodies also helps maintain unity of the minds and souls for married couples. Experiencing sexual pleasure with your spouse protects your marriage. In a society where the odds are stacked against happy marriages, the importance of joy, intimacy, and connection between spouses cannot be overstated. The sex life in marriage is a source of each of those elements and should be safeguarded. In uniting the body, mind, and spirit, spouses are reminded that they have united their lives.

While the intimate expression of love is unique and different to each couple, the foundations that allow for the most complete and wondrous sexual expression are the same for every couple.

Chapter 12
fRood to fRood free

"You are free to choose your own way of life, but you are not free to choose the results." - Dr. Herbert Shelton

Becoming fRood free is a process. There will be bumpy times, sacrifice, and moments that make you think it is not worth the change. It is and there are a few keys to remember throughout the journey.

1. <u>Attitude is going to make or break the transition.</u> Initially, you or your family may be unhappy about the giving up fRood or time in front of the tv. For this reason, you need to be extremely clear on why you are doing this. Whether it is for health, happiness, or a better sex life, write it down and read it every morning. Then get excited about where this new lifestyle is going to take you. Children will be more willing to accepting to live fRood free when they see it leads to happiness around them. I know this from personal experience. When I have had the freedom, I have been able to change the diets of families that I work for. Kids who previously would not touch

vegetables were suddenly willing to at least try whatever I put in front of them. This had nothing to with consequences or bribes, and everything to do with my attitude. the children would watch the way I ate and ask questions. I would answer and always be sure to comment on how good the food I ate makes me feel. Then I would ask if they wanted to try it. At first the answer would be an immediate no, but over time, hesitation appeared before the no, and then one day I would get a yes. Now that didn't mean the kids always liked what they tried. Whenever a child tried something new or ate a healthy food, I would get excited and give out lots of high fives.

As you can see, it is simply a matter of giving kids something better than sugar. And love, attention, and fun are those very things. Children crave love more than anything, so by substituting it for sugar, your children will not only accept the changes, but you will notice food becoming less of a priority to them. Their focus will stop revolving around what they get to eat next and will instead be geared to what they get to do next with you. The shift from food being a form of entertainment to fuel for entertaining yourself is one the most important attitude adjustments that you can teach your child. And it can be done by example.

When I moved back to Ohio and started writing this book, my house was full of men, who didn't particularly like to cook and weren't very focused on nutrition. When I took over grocery shopping and made it my mission to improve their nutrition, they weren't all thrilled. The fact that sugary cereal, junk bagels, junk yogurt, and junk granola bars suddenly were not filling the pantry shelves did not impress certain people. But as I substituted smoothies, muffins, and home cooked meals, they were less resistant. And the resistance crumbled when I added back massages to my arsenal.

2. <u>Get your kids involved in the process</u>. There are so many things that kids can do to help out in the kitchen. Washing vegetables and fruit, setting the table, and packing lunches are all chores kids can help out with. Use the transition to begin to teach your kids the importance of eating healthy. Showing them how to do so sets them up for success in life. If they learn now, they can avoid so much pain later. Eating

healthy will be a habit for them when they are living on their own and they will appreciate that you taught them that. There is a much better chance that they will not deal with fRood addiction when they are older if you teach them proper nutrition when they are young. It is extremely important that you do teach them why eating healthy is so important and not just to feed them healthy food. If they don't know why they are supposed to eat in a certain manner, they will much more easily start eating fRood when they are in charge out of their own health.

Here are some ways that I have taught kids about nutrition without them feeling like they are sitting in a classroom.

- Incorporate it into grace. "Thank you God for these awesome sunflower seeds, that are going to help Johnny in his football game today since they have lots of Vitamin E, which can help you play longer because it helps your cells get lots of oxygen."
- Explain why you eat the things that you do. "I'm eating this red pepper because its packed with vitamin B6, which keeps me happy and energetic so that I can play and laugh with you!"
- Include it in coloring time and activity. Turn it into a game. Ask them to draw the coolest thing that eating spinach does for you.

The ways of teaching your kids about nutrition are endless. I have seen kids get into it time and time again. It is a much better route them having them study nutrition labels to make sure there is not too much fat, sugar, or sodium in whatever they are about to eat. They don't have to worry about those things if they are eating food! It is also a better approach to have kids focus on the benefits of filling their diets with food than having their focus be on limiting their intake of fRood.

Sitting down with your children at dinner and eating that broccoli with them (on the count of three: ready, 1,2,3) and smiling and explaining that the broccoli is going to help them become big and strong like their dad is going to yield much more positive results than simply dishing it out and commanding that it be eaten because it is good for them.

Make it a family effort. Kids can help in the kitchen. And it can be fun. It's a chance to teach your kids while laughing and working with them. And then you get to enjoy eating with them. Use meals to bond with, to engage in lively and fun conversation with, and to get to know your children. As you are changing the menu, sit down and eat with your children. If breakfast is strawberries and almonds, initiate a conversation about the texture of the almond, about where almonds come from, about how you think God came up with the idea for strawberries. Stimulate your children's imaginations and get ready for some hilarious and interesting insights from them. Take time to enjoy your children because they can sense it and it will keep you close through the years. And when children know that you are interested in their opinions and thoughts, they will time and time again wow you with their intricate and unique personalities.

3. <u>Laugh…. a lot.</u> Be aware that there are definitely going to be bumps in the road. As more cooking occurs and less fRood makes its way into your children's mouths, there is going to be complaining at one point or another. They won't always like what you make. While I know that it can be hard to feel like you've spent valuable time making something that your family doesn't seem to appreciate, it happens. When I have a food disaster or spend time making something that is less than a hit, I chalk it up to practice and then I just think about one of my older brother's garlic stew and laugh.

He had just bought a crock pot and decided that following a recipe was not necessary. So, he placed all his ingredients into the pot in the morning, turned it on and left for the day. By the time I arrived home from work that evening, I could smell garlic as soon as I got out of my car. It was literally wafting out of the apartment in pungent waves. Neighbors were wondering if some sort of garlic stink bomb had been dropped. I opened the door to find our other roommate exiting. He had just gotten home as well but decided he was going out for dinner. I went straight to my room and locked myself in there. It didn't help. When my brother finally arrived I found out that he had used two entire bulbs of garlic instead a couple of cloves (about 20x the right amount). I'm still laughing as I write this.

That story shows how misadventures in the kitchen can be funny. Humor will make the transition much easier and will help create great memories. They just may not smell or taste so great.

When I was in fifth grade, three of my brothers and I were attending a very small school at the time where there was no talking permitted during lunch. One morning when he was on lunch duty, a certain brother was feeling mischievous. At lunch that day, I unpacked my food and proceeded to take a bite of my sandwich. The most foreign taste hit my tongue and I couldn't bite all the way through the sandwich. When I peeled off the top piece of bread, I saw layers of dried black seaweed. I gagged and snuck a glance over at the saboteur, who was silently snickering, trying to keep from laughing out loud to avoid getting in trouble. I wanted to throw my sandwich at him but swore vengeance and snuck a glance at my other brothers instead, who looked bewildered and unpleased. While I'm still trying to think of an adequate prank to pay him back for that stunt, the hours spent laughing about it made the seaweed sandwich my favorite lunch from childhood. It's even funnier because I love the taste of seaweed now. So much so that there is a running joke in my family that one day I'm going to run out of seaweed and go jump in the pond and fight with the fishes over the algae. As if!

The bottom line is that eating healthy can be made fun and funny. The closer your family becomes and the more fun you have together, the more willing kids will be to eat whatever you put in front of them.

4. Week by week. Transitions like this don't happen overnight. The best approach is to make a game plan that goes week by week. Here is one example. It may not be quite right for your family, but you can use it as a base model.

Week 1: Cut out processed foods that contain sugar and make your own desserts. Start out the morning with fruit.

Week 3: Cut out juice, dressings, and marinades. Eat at least 3 (2 raw) servings of vegetables a day.

Week 5: Cut out all refined sugar and flours from the diet. Replace with dates and whole grain flours.

Week 7: Cut out all processed snacks and replace with raw nuts and seeds.

Week 9: Cut out all remaining fRood from the diet and try to eat a rainbow each day.

5. <u>Nutrition outside the home</u>. As you improve the way your children eat at home, you may want to improve what they are eating elsewhere. Look no further than school. Packing lunches is the best option because it doesn't give your child money to spend on junk instead of lunch. Which happens all the time! In my five years of nannying, I was simply astounded at how much sugar was doled out at children's schools. Besides the vending machines and desserts at lunch, kids would come home with candy, sugary snacks, and even pop from the teachers. Talk to your child's teachers, talk to other parents, to the principle, or at the PTA about getting sugar out of the school. Children should be learning about the harmful effects of sugar at school, not having it handed out to them.

Transition Activities

- Smoothie tasting. Have your kids take turns making smoothies without the others watching and then have the other family members guess what ingredients were used. I have more fun doing this with one of my brothers than you can imagine- we get so into it you might think that we are wine tasting.
- Create your own grace- as you lead it you can simultaneously thank God for the nutrients in your food and teach your children about the wonders of nutrition.
- Teach your children about all the amazing things vitamins do by turning it into a game-challenge them to learn about a specific vitamin, mineral, ect and choose what they think its coolest function is and why and have them come up with a name for it based on what it does. You can also do this yourself with meals you serve them. Telling them sweet potatoes brightens and makes their skin glow is a way better reason to them than because its good for you or because I said so.

- Make you own nut butters- Much healthier than most selections available at the store-no hydrogenated oils, sugar, and you can make them raw. You can also make all different sorts- cashew butter, pecan butter,
- Rainbow grocery cart- while in the produce department with your kids have them fill the cart with roy g. biv (with a special focus on the g(reens) of course.
- DIY trail mix- buy a bunch of different ingredients for trail mix and spend an hour on a saturday with your kids letting them each make their own version... which is then theirs for the snacking. they will love it. as a kid who used to plow through snacks the day the arrived in order to get some before it disappeared, I know that kids appreciate having things that are theirs.
- Gardening- if you are into gardening at all.... get your kids involved. they will love it and it will be a special memory and connection that you share.
- making ice cream or juice popsicles with real fruit in them
- Let your kids plan out a meal and then help them make it- its a great way to bond and simultaneously teach them how to plan healthy meals
- Invent healthy substitutes- we all have snacks or foods that we love that we know aren't healthy choices. I discovered though that when I took the time to think about it, I could create my own healthier versions of those things.
- Berry/apple picking. In the summer and fall go pick your own. check out pickyourown.org to find farms near you.   Prices are normally pretty good and its a great way be on your feet and out in nature.
- Spa days- this is a great activity to do with your daughters- you can use leftovers (dregs from almond milk. avocados past their peak ect) to make your own hair masks, face masks, foot soaks, ect). Not only is a lot cheaper than going to an actual spa, but you are actually putting nutrients into your body that will make your skin glow)
- Include your kids in everyday activities that you do anyway. Example. My driveway was 1/4 of a mile long when I was a kid. Every sunday I would get up even earlier than I had to for church so that I could walk down to get the paper with my dad. I loved it.

Kids desperately want one on one time with parents--- and you have the ability to make that time special no matter what the activity is (shucking fresh corn during the summer, making homemade applesauce)

- Farmer's markets- yes they can be expensive... but if you trade in eating out for a weekly trip with the family, it can fit in the budget and it is also a great way to eat what is in season and local, i.e.... what is more nutritious because it was not picked before it was ripe, shipped halfway around the world, and then sprayed with chemicals to induce ripening.
- Contests in the kitchen- have mini cook offs where you come up with a challenge for your kids and then they create delicacies and submit them for judging.
- make your own dressing/sauce. Put out all different ingredients (oil, spices, cilantro, juices (lemon, whatever else) and let each kid make their own sauce that they can then use for salads and veggie dip at snack time. It's fun and they even come up up with fun names for their dressing and label them
- Sprouts- Sprouting seeds is not very time consuming, is very cheap, and is fun for kids because they can see the process unfold right in front of them. You can have a mini garden right in your kitchen Tiny little seeds become green sprouts over the course of a few days, which are chalked full of both nutrients and enzymes. Then they can be thrown into salads, stir fries, or put on sandwiches.

Chapter 13
The $avings of Health

Eating food instead of fRood will save you time, money, and sanity.

Time

There are three major ways that changing your family's diet will save time. A healthy diet reduces sickness, reduces time spent on issues in your family caused by diet, and increases energy and therefore efficiency. Feeding your family food will drastically reduce sickness in your home. It saves you time spent at home with sick children and trips to the doctors office.

A healthy diet means happier and better behaved children. It saves you time spent on homework, dealing with temper tantrums, at family counseling, nagging, and even looking for lost things. I have noticed that kids with poor diets have a much harder time keeping track of their belongings than children with healthy diets. Obviously personality plays a part in this, but without a doubt, diet also plays a role. This is because kids with diets comprised of food can think more clearly and track back in their minds to figure out where they left things. fRood fed children, on the other hand, who often deal with low blood sugar, are always at a loss for how to find their missing items. They cannot think back to the last place the remember putting said item because it is all a haze. They cannot concentrate or remember clearly.

A major hang up that holds people back from transitioning to a healthy lifestyle is the notion that it takes too much time. There is no time to cook healthy meals. There is no time to be physically active. There is simply no time. By having your family all pitch in and work together to create healthy meals and then being physically active together, everyone has increased energy and efficiency. This means that homework and chores take less time.

The fact is that changing your lifestyle to incorporate healthier habits does not add time. First of all, any unhealthy habits present in your family WILL cost you time. It costs time when your children get sick, it costs times because you are not functioning as efficiently as you can when you are healthy, and it costs time off your life in the future. When your energy is low, whether it is due to poor digestion, depression, or fatigue, you are not operating anywhere near the potential you possess if you were to treat your body the way it needs to be treated. There is absolutely no way around the time costs that accompany poor standards of health. When you are eating foods that nourish your mind and body, you have more energy, you can accomplish more in a less amount of time, and you WILL be happier. The same goes for your children. With proper nutrition, their concentration, energy, and attitude will all increase. That leads to shorter time spent doing homework, less nagging for them to accomplish chores, better performance at sports, and less pouting.

The best way to conserve time is to combine the elements of health with family time. That means that meal time including preparation should include more than just you mom. Once your kids are old enough, work out tasks that they can help you with. Washing vegetables, setting the table, and doing dishes are all tasks that your kids can be involved in. And when you work together it makes it that much more rewarding to sit down together as a family and enjoy a meal together.

Instead of joining a gym and then never having the time to go there, get your physical activity by playing with your kids. Tag, kickball, running from the tickle monster are all activities that provide you and your kids exercise, fun, and quality family time. By quality family time I mean activities through which you bond with your children. Time spent in front of the tv laughing has no comparison to the laughter that comes through play. Kids don't continually bring up how hard you laughed about this scene in such and such a movie the way the they do the time where you wiped out on your bum chasing them across the yard. Kids hunger for playtime WITH their parents. I know I did. And I still enjoy it. To get out and play tennis with my dad or play king of the raft with him and my brothers lifts my spirits unbelievably high. It makes me so sad when I see parents at parks, beaches, or homes who simply will not play with their children.

The excuse that you do not have time to get out and be physically active with your children is one that needs to be left at the front door as you exit. This is because exercise increases energy which leads to a more efficient you. And getting your kids outside to play also gets them ready for bed. Tucker your kids out. I went to bed as a kid at 7. And I did not argue. Not because I didn't want to be yelled at, but because I was happy to go to bed. I was tired from the day. I know lots of kids who don't go to bed until 10. So while it may seem like it takes too much time to be active with your kids, you get that time back later. Imagine that moms. It is 7:30 pm, your kids are asleep and you have..... time to yourself? Or time to spend with your husband? It is worth it... and as another bonus, you will sleep better to because you got some activity in your day.

I have watched parents struggle with their kids for hours and hours. Getting a four year old into pajamas, calming down an eight year old from a massive tantrum, reasoning with an angry ten year old, are all things that are connected to improper nutrition and take up massive amounts of time. Can you imagine how awesome it would be to sideline behavior like this? Think of how much less stressed you would be if homework time, bath time, and bed time were less like war zones and actually fun times full of laughter, learning, and connection. And I am telling you, it is not a fairy tale. I have seen the transition and the difference it makes in families. I have been on both sides of the fence and once you hop over it, you will know that you're on the greener side and never want to go back.

$

What is your family's health and happiness worth to you? Getting healthy and happy doesn't have be an added expense to your budget. First it is important to make the distinctions between food and fRood and then to decide that fRood no longer gets to take up shelf space in your food budget. It is also necessary to realize how fRood impacts the whole household budget.   fRood results in so much spending it's almost unbelievable.   Healthcare expenses top the list. Sickness, broken bones, disease, dental and psychological services are all impacted by fRood consumption.   The more fRood consumed in your family, the more money that has to be spent on healthcare. It is important to realize that the food budget is not the only part of the household budget that is impacted when it comes to choosing what to put into the grocery cart. If you redefine what qualifies as food, you will notice that it is suddenly much more affordable to buy healthy food.

1. fRood should not be part of your food budget. It is poisonous and would be better categorized with a budget for alcohol and cigarettes.
   a. If you are buying a box of sugary cereal for $3, there is nothing in that cereal that is real food-therefore it shouldn't be a part of your food budget.
2. Stop thinking about food costs in terms of price/pound. Consider it in nutrients/price.
   a. Calories from refined sugar, flours and grains, unhealthy oils, and GMOs should never count as food.
   b. While vegetables and fruits may not pack in many calories, they pack in the nutrients that you truly need. So while a pound of broccoli may not buy you as many calories as two items from the dollar menu, it buys you health and prevents you from a future heart attack.

3. Juice, soda, sports drinks, energy drinks, and designer coffee drinks should have no place in your food budget.

Eating food instead of fRood can prevent you from having to spend money on therapy for family counseling. There is so much mental distress and so many problems in marriages that are the results of malnutrition. All these issues can lead to thousands of dollars spent on psychologists when the root of the problem and the solution lie in what you are eating.

There are so many healthy foods out there that are so much cheaper than eating fRood. Beans, whole grains like oats and brown rice, whole grain flours, and sweet potatoes are all awesome for you and will not drain your bank account. Items that truly waste your money are things like pop, poptarts, pizza, and pastries. You are paying money for items that harm your family's health and harm your pocketbook now and will harm it again somewhere in the future.

Here is a change that would definitely result in more cash in your wallet. I see so many kids that drink milk (best case) or soda (worse case) instead of water at all meals. This is setting your child up with horrible habits for the rest of their life. And it is expensive. I was once nannying a two year old who was on the rebound from acid-reflux. All this child had ever drank in his bottle was juice. His mother was constantly worried that he didn't eat enough. I had slowly been taking the massive amounts of sugar out of his diet since I had started and then took him completely off juice. The dad came home one day, sidled over to the high chair, and was almost indignant that I had given his child water. "what is that you're drinking there... Is that water?" At which point he turned to me, "he's over all the burping and throwing up. You can give him juice again." I kept him drinking water and watched his appetite spike incredibly. He would be so hungry after a trip to the park or running around outside that he would eat anything I put in front of him. As soon as the mother got home from work, the first thing he had to say of course was, "I want juice!" But he never asked for it while I was there and would comment how good water was. He might not have really enjoyed it, but he watched me drink water all day and would copy me. If I put the glass to my lips, so did he.   Another great example of how kids learn through example. They want to be just like those they look up to.

Sanity

Choosing food over fRood is going to keep you from losing your mind.   It will save you from thoughts like, "Is this all there is is?", "Why bother?", and "This is not how I envisioned my life". The point is that food can rescue you and your family! It can save you from so much struggle, so many problems, and so much unhappiness. It really does have that much power! Eating food will allow you to achieve the hopes and dreams you have for your family and help you stay sane along the way.

Chapter 14
fRood Free Recipes

* Most of these recipes do not qualify as excellent food combinations. However, they are a step up from the products that they mimic. The awesome sauce does qualify as an awesome combo!

Staples
Date Puree- dates are an amazing fruit. I have completely eliminated sugar from my house and use dates to sweeten everything from baked goods to hot cocoa. They are packed with vitamins, fiber, and potassium.
Simply take dates, and pour just enough almond milk or even water to cover them. Let them sit for a few hours and then put them in a food processor or blender and puree them. Refrigerate the puree.

Almond Milk- cheaper to make than to buy, it is an awesome substitution for regular milk in all kinds of recipes

Rinse and soak ½ cup of almonds overnight in water with a ¼ tsp of salt. Rinse again and then either peel the almonds or not, before placing in a blender with 4 cups of water and blending for at least two minutes. Strain through a nut milk bag if you want a smooth consistency or leave the dregs for fiber. Wala! You have just become a milk maid (or man) and have a delicious and healthy almond milk.

<u>Sprouts</u>- There is a plethora of seeds that can be acquired online or in health food stores that you can grow in a few days right in your kitchen. All you have to do is soak them over night and then rinse them twice a day. Minimal work and cost with a maximum payout for your health. Clover, alfalfa, broccoli, and radish are just a few of the choices. There are containers you can buy or just use mason jars and cheesecloth.

Awesome Sauce

Oranges, avocado, and some sort of frozen berry- amounts used vary by taste and preference but each smoothie in my house contains about 1 large orange, 1/2 of a small avocado, and 1 cup of frozen berries. Prep- layer orange at the bottom of the blender, followed by avocado, and the frozen berries on top. Blend away and enjoy.
*Using whole fruit is much better than juice because it is fresh, full of fiber, and much better for stable blood sugar levels. Again, it comes back to keeping foods in as natural a state as possible for your best possible health. You can also add in spinach, cucumbers, or even kale without your youngster's becoming suspicious. Or you can use kale and dip it into the smoothies. Some of my younger brothers and I do this and its delicious!

<u>Chocolate Milk</u>- Can be enjoyed warm or cold

8 oz almond milk (or any other nut milk of choice)
dash of vanilla extract
1 TBS cocoa
2 TBS date puree

Mix the ingredients in a blender and then enjoy cold or warm it up on the stove for hot cocoa

Awesome Orbs
One pound of pitted dates
½ cup coconut oil
½ cup of coconut manna- you can buy or prepare yourself
¼ cup of cocoa
2 tsp of vanilla extract

Throw it all into a food processor and press the on button.
Form into little orbs- according to you size preference and place on a
wax sheet covering a cookie sheet
Refrigerate and enjoy

Nutty ice cream- It's a perfect substitute for ice cream
Two cups almond milk- store bought or home made
1/4-1/3 cup of nut butter (peanut, almond, cashew, pecan, ect)
2 tsp of flavoring extract (vanilla, maple, whatever strikes your fancy)
8 medium/large pitted dates
dash of salt
Prep- let the dates soak in the the almond milk for about 6 hours.
place in blender and blend
add in flavor extract, salt, and nut butter and blend some more
pour into shallow containers and freeze
Enjoy

Nutmegger- when my younger brothers need energy for a soccer
game or some other activity, these bars provide the fuel. They taste
similar to cookie dough
Choice of peanuts, cashews, pecans, almonds, or combo
Dates- ¼ to ⅓ of the amount of nut
dash of vanilla

Throw in food processor and then mold into bars. Or pretend it is
cookie dough and eat it with a spoon.

<u>Oatmeal bakes</u>- this can be made into almost any flavor you want. The base ingredients are:

1 cup of oatmeal
1/4 cup of date puree

From there, you can add in the ingredients to make whatever sort you want. Some of my family's favorites are:

Raspberry streusel- 2 TBS of butter and 1/2 a cup of fresh/frozen raspberries

Banana nut-2 TBS of butter, a mashed banana, some cinnamon, and some walnuts (use only 1/8 of date puree for this option)

Chocolate PB- 2 TBS of peanut butter, 2 TBS of cocoa, and 1 tsp of vanilla

Apply oats- 2 TBS of cashew butter/coconut oil/or butter, cinnamon, and 1/4 cup applesauce or 1/4 chopped apple (use only and 1/8th a cup of date puree if using applesauce)

Combine all ingredients and cook in the oven at 370* for 15 minutes and then set it to broil for 3 minutes if you want a nice crisp crust on top.

You could also make coconut, pumpkin, or other berry versions of this. Just experiment and see what you and your family like. It doesn't take very long to prepare and I guarantee that your kids will love starting fall and winter days off with a nice warm oat bake. And you will love that your kid has not filled himself with captain crunch before school.

<u>Wholy Grain Pancakes</u>

1 Cup Whole Grain flour (oat, spelt, buckwheat)
1/2 Cup Rolled Oats
1/3 Cup Ground Flax
1 and a 1/3 cup buttermilk
1 tsp baking powder
1 tsp baking soda

1/2 tsp salt
2 eggs

Combine flour, oats, flax, baking powder, baking soda, and salt together
Beat egg and add along with buttermilk until blended
Heat up a pan and let the pancakes sizzle!

Bowl to Mouth Brownie Batter
Cashew butter
date paste
cocoa powder
dash of vanilla extract
Mix together in equal amounts (except for vanilla) and enjoy ray

Mine Mine Muffins-

2 cups of whole grain flour
2 tsp baking powder
2 eggs
1/2 tsp salt
3 TBS melted butter
2/3 cup of date puree

now for the add ins
raspberry- add 2 cups of frozen raspberries
coffee cake-add 2 tsp vanilla and make this mixture(1/2 cup date puree, 2 tsp cinnamon, and 1/2 cup of walnuts or pecans). Place half of the batter into the muffin pans, evenly spread the mixture on top and then cover with the rest of the batter.

combine all ingredients, pour into greased muffin pan, and cook for 20 minutes at 350*

Sweet Potato Fries- So much more delicious and healthy than your standard fry and could be part of a disappearing act they vanish so quickly.

As many potatoes as you desire
Oil (avoid soy)
spices you like (salt, pepper, cayenne it you like them spicy, cajun for a twist)

Peel the potatoes, slice, and toss them in a bowl with a generous drizzle of oil and spices.
Spread them out on a baking sheet and put them into the oven at 400* for 20-30 minutes, depending on how you like them cooked.

Hummingbird Cake- the new every occasion cake.

2 ¼ cups whole grain flour
2 ½ cups baking powder
1 tsp salt
1 ½ cups date puree
2 ripe bananas
1 cup canned, strained pineapple (in juice, not syrup)
3 large eggs (beaten)
½ cup butter or vegetable oil.

Sift flour, baking powder, and salt together.
Blend date puree, bananas, and pineapple together
Add the eggs and butter/oil to the flour mixture.
Add fruit blend.
Pour into a greased bunt pan.
Cook for 50 min at 350* or until a wood pick comes out clean when inserted into the center of the cake.

Salsa-

tomatoes- 3 medium
jalepenos- this depends on how much you like spice and how hot the
jalepenos are
scallions- one bunch
onion- one small
garlic-3 cloves
lime- juice from one
black pepper

chop it up or throw it in a food processor and then enjoy. Personally, I
like to eat it like soup or use cabbage to scoop it up. My family will
eat a gallon of this stuff in one day in the summer!

*Throwing some avocado in there is also delicious and increases your
body's absorption of the ninja nutrients it contains.

Chapter 15
I Dare You

I dare you to go fRood free. I double dog dare you! If you doubt any of the ancient pearls of wisdom I have laid out in this book, I dare you to try and prove me wrong. Don't quote flimsy trials or clinical studies to me. Go fRood free for one month and let your results be the proof. Or just try incorporating a couple concepts into your life. Consider this book a buffet table and pile your plate with the ideas that you feel will have a beneficial impact on you and your family.

Whether you want to wake up in the morning and feel stoked about getting out of bed, have a closer knit family, super charge your sex life, or tackle a specific health issue, ditching fRood is the place to start.

During your dare, here are some guiding principles to focus on:

1. Eat a rainbow every day- and find the health that is more precious than gold.
2. Have some sprouts and raw nut milk each day.

3. Take time to play each day
4. Refined sugar sucks the life, vitality, and youth out of you- give it the axe
5. Minimize wheat, soy, and dairy
6. Separate proteins and starches and simplify your meals
7. When in doubt, consider what the Chief of Nutrition would think.

Bibliography

- Abrahamson, E. M., and A.W. Pezet. Body, Mind, and Sugar. New York: Henry Holt and Company, 1951.

- Airaola, Paavo. Sex & Nutrition. New York: Charter Communications Inc., 1970.

- Biehler, Henry. Food is Your Best Medicine. New York: Ballantine Books, 1982.

- Blaine, Tom. Mental Health Through Nutrition. New York: The Citadel Press, 1969.

- Connors, Keith. Feeding the brain: how foods affect children. New York: Plenum Press, 1989.

- Evans, Isabelle. Sugar, Sex, and Sanity. New York: Carlton Press Inc., 1970.

- Haas, Elson, and Buck Levin. Staying Healthy with Nutrition. New York: Ten Speed Press, 2006.

- Hurdle, Frank. Low Blood Sugar: A Doctor's Guide to its Effective Control. West Nyack: Parker Publishing Company Inc., 1969

- Jensen, Bernard. Dr. Jensen's Guide to Better Bowel Care. Garden City Park: Avery Publishing Group Inc., 1999.

- Jensen, Bernard. Dr. Jensen's Nutrition Handbook: a daily regimen for healthy living. Chicago: Keats Publishing, 200

- Jensen, Bernard. Love, Sex, and Nutrition. Garden City Park: Avery Publishing Group Inc., 1988.

- Martin, Clement. Low Blood Sugar The Hidden Menace of Hypoglycemia. New York: Fireside, 1992.

- Null, Gary, et al. Food Combining Handbook. New York: Pyramid Health, 1977.

- Rodale, J.I.. Natural Health, Sugar, and the Criminal Mind. New York: Pyramid Books, 1968.

- Shelton, Herbert. Food Combining...made Easy. San Antonio: Dr. Shelton's Health School, 1951.

- Stitt, Barbara. Food and Behavior. Manitowoc: Natural Press, 1997.

- Tessler, Gordon. Sex, Nutrition, and You. San Diego: Better Health Publishers, 1986

- Watson, George. Nutrition and Your Mind. New York: Harper & Row, Publishers, 1972.

- Weller, Patti. The Power of Nutrient Dense Food. El Cajon: Deerpath Publishing Company, 2007.

- Yudkin, John. Pure, White and Deadly. New York: Viking Penguin Inc, 1986.

www.ingramcontent.com/pod-product-compliance
Lightning Source LLC
Chambersburg PA
CBHW050357280326
41933CB00010BA/1496